STUDY GUIDE FOR
Pharmacology *for* Health Professionals

STUDY GUIDE FOR
Pharmacology
for Health
Professionals

Jean Zorko

Assistant Professor
General Studies Division
Science Department
Stark State College of Technology
Canton, Ohio

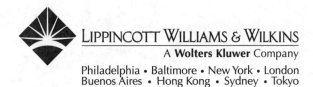

LIPPINCOTT WILLIAMS & WILKINS
A **Wolters Kluwer** Company

Philadelphia • Baltimore • New York • London
Buenos Aires • Hong Kong • Sydney • Tokyo

Acquisitions Editor: John Goucher
Managing Editor: Kevin C. Dietz
Marketing Manager: Hilary Henderson
Production Editor: Christina Remsberg
Compositor: Maryland Composition
Printer: Victor Graphics

Printed in the United States of America

Library of Congress Cataloging-in-Publication Data

The publishers have made every effort to trace the copyright holders for borrowed material. If they have inadvertently overlooked any, they will be pleased to make the necessary arrangements at the first opportunity.

To purchase additional copies of this book, call our customer service department at **(800) 638-3030** or fax orders to **(301) 824-7390**. International customers should call **(301) 714-2324**.

Visit Lippincott Williams & Wilkins on the Internet: http://www.LWW.com. Lippincott Williams & Wilkins customer service representatives are available from 8:30 am to 6:00 pm, EST.

05 06 07 08 09
1 2 3 4 5 6 7 8 9 10

Table of Contents
Study Guide for Pharmacology for Health Professionals

1 General Principles of Pharmacology

I. MATCHING

Match the term from Column A with the correct definition from Column B.

COLUMN A

_____ 1. additive drug reaction

_____ 2. antagonist

_____ 3. agonist

_____ 4. controlled substance

_____ 5. hypersensitivity

_____ 6. pharmaceutic phase

_____ 7. pharmacokinetics

_____ 8. polypharmacy

_____ 9. receptor

_____ 10. teratogen

COLUMN B

A. The taking of numerous drugs that can potentially react with one another.
B. Any substance that causes abnormal development of the fetus.
C. Drugs with a high potential for abuse that are controlled by special regulations.
D. A specialized macromolecule that binds to the drug molecule, altering the function of the cell and producing the therapeutic response.
E. Activities occurring within the body after a drug is administered.
F. Being allergic to a drug.
G. A drug that binds with a receptor to produce a therapeutic response.
H. A drug that joins with a receptor to prevent the action of an agonist at that receptor.
I. A reaction that occurs when the combined effect of two drugs is equal to the sum of each drug given alone.
J. The dissolution of the drug.

II. MATCHING

Match the item in Column A with the correct definition from Column B.

COLUMN A

_____ 1. Pure Food and Drug Act 1906

_____ 2. Harrison Narcotic Act 1914

_____ 3. Pure Food, Drug, and Cosmetic Act 1938

_____ 4. Controlled Substance Act 1970

_____ 5. Comprehensive Drug Abuse Prevention and Control Act 1970

_____ 6. Drug Enforcement Agency (DEA)

_____ 7. Food and Drug Administration (FDA)

_____ 8. Dietary Supplement Health and Education Act (DSHEA)

_____ 9. Orphan Drug Act 1983

_____ 10. Investigational New Drug (IND)

COLUMN B

A. Chief federal agency responsible for enforcing the Controlled Substances Act.
B. Agency responsible for approving new drugs and monitoring drugs for adverse or toxic reactions.
C. Law that gives the FDA control over the manufacture and sale of drugs, food, and cosmetics.
D. First law that regulated the sale of narcotic drugs.
E. Regulates the manufacture, distribution, and dispensation of drugs with a potential for abuse.
F. First attempt by the U.S. government to regulate and control the manufacture, distribution, and sale of drugs.
G. Title II of the Comprehensive Drug Abuse Prevention and Control Act which deals with control and enforcement of the Act.

H. Act that defines herbs, vitamins, minerals, amino acids, and other natural supplements and permits general health claims as long as a disclaimer is present.

I. Encourages the development and marketing of products used to treat rare diseases.

J. The clinical testing phase of drug approval by the FDA.

III. TRUE/FALSE

Indicate whether each statement is True (T) or False (F).

_____ 1. A New Drug Application (NDA) is submitted immediately following Phase II of the clinical testing portion of the IND status.

_____ 2. The accelerated approval of drugs by the FDA seeks to make lifesaving investigational drugs available for healthcare providers to administer in early Phase I and II clinical trials.

_____ 3. The compassionate access program allows drugs to be given free of charge to patients in financial need.

_____ 4. Legend drugs can be prescribed by any healthcare provider.

_____ 5. Prescriptions for controlled substances must be written in ink, include the name and address of the patient, and the DEA number of the healthcare provider.

_____ 6. All drugs taken by mouth, except liquids, go through three phases: the pharmaceutic phase, the pharmacokinetic phase, and the pharmacodynamic phase.

_____ 7. The absorption of a drug is the process that refers to the activities involving the drug within the body after it is administered.

_____ 8. All drugs produce more than one effect on the body.

_____ 9. An allergic reaction to a drug occurs because the patient's immune system views the drug as an antibody.

_____ 10. Drug toxicity can be reversible or irreversible.

_____ 11. A pharmacogenetic disorder is a genetically caused abnormal response to a normal dose of a drug.

_____ 12. Herbs and nutritional supplements are "natural products" and therefore many individuals incorrectly assume they have no adverse effects.

IV. MULTIPLE CHOICE

Circle the letter of the best answer.

1. The pre-FDA phase of drug development includes _____.
   a. in vitro testing
   b. development of a promising drug
   c. testing using animal and human cells
   d. testing using live animals
   e. all of the answers are correct

2 and 3. The FDA phase of drug development requires the manufacturer of the drug to apply first for (2)_____, and then after three phases of clinical testing to apply for a (3)_____.
   a. clinical trial phase I
   b. IND
   c. NDA
   d. clinical trial phase II
   e. clinical trial phase III

4. The MedWatch system allows healthcare professionals to _____.
   a. track drug use by patient
   b. obtain pharmacy records of patients
   c. monitor prescriptions written by a physician
   d. report observations of serious adverse drug reactions anonymously
   e. contact government officials about insurance fraud

5. The Orphan Drug Program allows manufacturers to produce drugs that treat rare disorders; in exchange, the manufacturer may receive _____.
   a. grants
   b. tax incentives
   c. protocol assistance by the FDA
   d. 7 years of exclusive production rights for the drug involved
   e. all of the answers are correct

6. A _____ is a drug that the FDA has designated to be potentially harmful unless its use is supervised by a licensed healthcare provider.
   a. controlled substance
   b. prescription drug
   c. nonprescription drug
   d. legend drug
   e. answers b and d are correct

7. The Drug Enforcement Agency (DEA) _____.
   a. is under the U.S. Department of Justice
   b. enforces the Controlled Substances Act of 1970
   c. requires compliance by all healthcare workers
   d. can punish those who fail to comply by imprisonment
   e. all of the answers are correct

8. Pregnancy Category D drugs, whether prescription or nonprescription, _____.
   a. have a risk that cannot be ruled out
   b. have controlled studies that show no risk
   c. have positive evidence of risk to the human fetus
   d. are contraindicated in pregnancy
   e. none of the answers are correct

9. Pharmacokinetics refers to _____.
   a. absorption
   b. excretion
   c. distribution
   d. metabolism
   e. all of the answers are correct

10. The therapeutic level of a drug is the level at which _____.
    a. toxic symptoms may develop
    b. the drug is pharmacologically inactive
    c. the drug is effective
    d. the liver biotransforms the drug
    e. occurs directly after administration

11. Drugs whose action alters the cellular environment act to _____.
    a. change the physical environment
    b. change the chemical environment
    c. change both the physical and chemical environment
    d. change the cellular genetics
    e. change the drug action itself

12. The number of receptor sites available at a target site can _____.
    a. influence the effects of a drug
    b. change as a person ages

c. allow more potent drugs to be used
d. keep other drugs from acting
e. be chemically altered

13. Allergic or hypersensitivity reactions _____.
    a. usually begin to occur after more than one dose of a drug
    b. occur because the patient's immune system sees the drug as a foreign substance
    c. must be reported to the healthcare provider
    d. may occur within minutes after the drug is given
    e. all of the answers are correct

14. When a patient develops a tolerance to a drug, _____.
    a. they have a decreased response to the drug
    b. they will require an increase in dosage to achieve the desired effect
    c. it is an indicator of drug dependence
    d. the patient's body does not metabolize and excrete the drug before the next dose is given
    e. answers a, b, and c are correct

15. Drug interactions may occur _____.
    a. between two drugs
    b. between oral drugs and food
    c. answers a and b are correct
    d. between IV drugs and liquids
    e. often in young adults

16. A patient's response to a drug may be influenced by which of the following factors?
    a. disease
    b. age
    c. weight
    d. gender
    e. all of the answers are correct

17. The route of administration of a drug may influence a patient's drug response. The route order of response from most rapid to least rapid is _____.
    a. IV, IM, SC, oral
    b. IM, SC, oral, IV
    c. SC, oral, IV, IM
    d. oral, IM, SC, IV
    e. none of the answers are correct

18. The route of administration which results in the slowest drug action is _____.
    a. oral
    b. intravenous
    c. subcutaneous
    d. intramuscular
    e. transdermal

V. RECALL FACTS

Indicate which of the following statements are facts with an F. If the statement is not a fact, leave the line blank.

About Toxic Reactions/Levels

_____ 1. Can occur when drugs are administered in large doses

_____ 2. Some reactions are immediate while others may not be seen for months

_____ 3. Can be reversible or irreversible

_____ 4. Patients always know when a toxic reaction is going to occur

_____ 5. Can occur in recommended doses

_____ 6. Only licensed healthcare providers need to know the signs and symptoms of toxicity

About Herbal Therapy

_____ 1. Are regulated by the FDA

_____ 2. Cannot be sold or promoted as drugs in the United States

_____ 3. Are classified as dietary or nutritional supplements

_____ 4. Is widely taught in medical schools across the United States

_____ 5. Must have a disclaimer on the label that states that the supplements are not FDA approved

_____ 6. Can be important complementary or alternative therapy to drugs

About Controlled Substances

_____ 1. Have a high potential for abuse

_____ 2. May cause physical or psychological dependence

_____ 3. Prescriptions for these drugs cannot be filled more than 6 months after the prescription was written

_____ 4. Prescriptions for these drugs cannot be refilled more than five times.

_____ 5. Are the largest category of drugs

_____ 6. Are categorized in five schedules, C-I through C-V

About Drug Half-Life

_____ 1. 98% of drugs are eliminated in five to six half-lives

_____ 2. Increases with liver or kidney disease

_____ 3. Is the same for the same drug in most people

_____ 4. Can be altered by changing the dose

_____ 5. Is based on the frequency of administration

_____ 6. Is the time required for the body to eliminate 50% of the drug

VI. FILL IN THE BLANK

Fill in the blanks using words from the list below.

cellular	small
public	2–10
psychological	pharmacokinetics
8–12	physical
immediate	generic

1. The three phases of clinical testing of a new drug can last anywhere from _____ years.

2. _____ dependency is a compulsive need to use a substance repeatedly to avoid mild to severe withdrawal symptoms.

3. _____ dependency is a compulsion to use a substance to obtain a pleasurable experience.

4. In hospitals or other agencies that dispense controlled substances, scheduled drugs are counted every _____ hours.

5. Enteric coated drugs do not disintegrate until they reach the _____ intestine.

6. Most drugs act on the body by altering _____ function.

7. Changes that occur with aging affect the _____ of a drug.

8. The National Center for Complementary and Alternative Medicine (NCCAM) disseminates information to the _____.

9. Anaphylactic shock is a serious allergic drug reaction that requires _____ medical attention.

10. The _____ name of a drug is defined as the name given to a drug before it becomes official and may be used in all countries, by all manufacturers, and is not capitalized.

VII. LIST

List the requested number of items.

1. List the three categories to which the FDA assigns a new drug.
   a. _____
   b. _____
   c. _____

2. List four items that *must* be on a prescription for a drug.
   a. _____
   b. _____
   c. _____
   d. _____

3. List four items that *must* be on the product label of an OTC drug.
   a. _____
   b. _____
   c. _____
   d. _____

4. List the two phases that liquid and parenteral drugs go through in the body.
   a. _____
   b. _____

5. List the four activities that pharmacokinetics involves.

   a. _____
   b. _____
   c. _____
   d. _____

6. List the seven types of drug reactions in the body.
   a. _____
   b. _____
   c. _____
   d. _____
   e. _____
   f. _____
   g. _____

7. List the three effects of drug–drug interactions.
   a. _____
   b. _____
   c. _____

8. List the five schedules of controlled substances and give a brief definition.
   a. _____
   b. _____
   c. _____
   d. _____
   e. _____

9. List the four names that a drug may have.
   a. _____
   b. _____
   c. _____
   d. _____

10. List the five Pregnancy Categories and give a brief definition.
    a. _____
    b. _____
    c. _____
    d. _____
    e. _____

IX. CLINICAL APPLICATIONS

1. Mrs. C has recently discovered that she is pregnant. On her history and physical form you note that she takes many herbal remedies and dietary supplements as well as multiple over-the-counter medications. What might you suggest Mrs. C discuss with her healthcare provider?

2. Your overweight neighbor, knowing that you are in healthcare, wants to know why her prescription for antibiotics is the same strength as her elderly father who has kidney disease, but the other medication that they both take for cholesterol control have different dosages and schedules. What might you tell your neighbor in response?

I. MATCHING

Match the term from Column A with the correct definition from Column B.

COLUMN A

_____ 1. extravasation

_____ 2. inhalation

_____ 3. intradermal

_____ 4. intramuscular

_____ 5. intravenous

_____ 6. parenteral

_____ 7. subcutaneous

_____ 8. sublingual

_____ 9. transdermal

_____ 10. unit dose

COLUMN B

A. The escape of fluid from a blood vessel into surrounding tissues.

B. Route of administration in which the drug is injected into muscle tissue.

C. Route of administration in which the drug is injected into skin tissue.

D. Route of administration in which the drug is injected just below the layer of skin.

E. Route of administration in which the drug is absorbed through the skin from a patch.

F. Route of administration in which drug droplets, vapor, or gas is inhaled and absorbed through the mucous membranes of the respiratory tract.

G. Route of administration in which the drug is injected into a vein.

H. A single dose of a drug packaged ready for patient use.

I. Route of administration in which the drug is placed under the tongue for absorption.

J. A general term for drug administration in which the drug is injected inside the body.

II. TRUE/FALSE

Indicate whether each statement is True (T) or False (F).

_____ 1. A drug error is any occurrence that can cause a patient to receive the wrong dose, the wrong drug, the wrong route, or the drug at the wrong time.

_____ 2. A STAT order is an order to administer a drug as needed.

_____ 3. A standing order is an order written when a patient is to receive the prescribed drug on a regular basis.

_____ 4. An advantage of once-a-week dosing is that the patient who experiences mild adverse reactions would only have to experience them once a week rather than every day.

_____ 5. New OSHA guidelines help to reduce needlestick injuries among healthcare workers and others who handle medical sharps.

_____ 6. 80% of needlestick injuries can be prevented with the use of safe needle devices.

_____ 7. A subcutaneous injection places the drug into tissues below the muscle level.

_____ 8. The Z-track method of IM injection is used when a drug is highly irritating to subcutaneous tissues or may permanently stain the skin.

_____ 9. Whenever a drug is added to an IV fluid, the IV bag must have an attached label indicating the drug and dose added.

_____ 10. After an IV infusion is started, if either extravasation or infiltration occurs the infusion must be stopped and restarted in another vein.

_____ 11. The administration of drugs by the intradermal route usually requires special equipment.

_____ 12. Topical drugs act on the skin but are not absorbed through the skin.

III. MULTIPLE CHOICE

Circle the letter of the best answer.

1. When a drug error occurs, the healthcare worker should _____.
   a. wait to see if any adverse effects occur
   b. report the incident immediately
   c. not tell anyone so they do not get into trouble
   d. tell the patient not to worry
   e. none of these answers are correct

2. In a computerized dispensing system the _____.
   a. drug orders are filled and medications are dispensed to fill each patient's medication order for a 24-hour period
   b. drugs that are dispensed are automatically recorded in a computerized system
   c. a bar code scanner is used to record and charge routine and PRN drugs
   d. the drugs most frequently ordered are kept on the unit in containers in a designated medication room
   e. all of these methods are part of the computerized dispensing system

3. Healthcare professionals involved in drug administration should know _____.
   a. the reason the drug is used
   b. the drug's general actions and adverse reactions
   c. special precautions in administration
   d. normal dose ranges
   e. all of this information should be known

4. Oral route drug administration _____.
   a. is the most frequent route of administration
   b. rarely causes physical discomfort
   c. is relatively easy for patients who are alert and can swallow
   d. can use drug forms such as tablets, capsules, or liquids
   e. all of the answers are correct

5. A method of parenteral drug administration is _____.
   a. subcutaneous
   b. intramuscular
   c. intravenous
   d. intradermal
   e. all of the answers are correct

6. Parenteral routes of administration can include _____.
   a. intra-articular
   b. intralesional
   c. intra-arterial
   d. intracardiac
   e. all of the answers are correct

7. Drugs administered by the subcutaneous route _____.
   a. are absorbed more slowly than are intramuscular drugs
   b. are delivered into the tissues between the skin and the muscle
   c. can be given in large amounts (greater than 1 mL)
   d. are generally given in the upper arm, upper back, or upper abdomen
   e. answers a, b, and d are correct

8. Sites for the administration of intramuscular drugs are _____.
   a. deltoid muscle
   b. ventrogluteal muscle
   c. dorsogluteal muscle
   d. vastus lateralis muscle
   e. all of the answers are correct

9. Infusion controllers and infusion pumps are electronic infusion devices. The primary difference between the two is that _____.
   a. an infusion pump administers the infused drug under pressure, and an infusion controller does not add pressure
   b. an infusion pump administers the infused drug without added pressure, whereas an infusion controllers adds pressure
   c. both devices administer the drug under pressure; the difference is the amount of pressure used
   d. there is no difference; the two devices are the same
   e. none of these answers are correct

10. Intradermal drug administration _____.
    a. usually results in the formation of a wheal
    b. requires a 90° angle of needle insertion
    c. provides good results for allergy testing or local anesthesia
    d. requires a portal to be implanted in the skin
    e. answers a and c are correct

IV. RECALL FACTS

Indicate which of the following statements are Facts with an F. If the statement is not a fact, leave the line blank.

About IV Drug Administration

_____ 1. Are given directly into the blood by a needle inserted into a vein.

_____ 2. Drug action occurs almost immediately.

_____ 3. May be given slowly (>1 minute) or rapidly (<1 minute).

_____ 4. Can be delivered by an IV port or through a heparin lock.

About Transdermal Drug Administration

_____ 1. Allows the drug to be readily absorbed from the skin and have systemic effects.

_____ 2. Allows for a relatively constant blood concentration.

_____ 3. Increases the risk of toxicity.

_____ 4. The sites are rotated to prevent skin irritation.

_____ 5. Should have the site shaved of hair before administration.

_____ 6. Old patches are removed before a new dose is applied.

About After a Drug Is Administered

_____ 1. Is always documented as soon as possible.

_____ 2. The patient's response to the drug is monitored.

_____ 3. The patient's vital signs are not taken until several hours after the drug is administered.

_____ 4. IV flow rate, site used, or problems with administration are recorded.

_____ 5. Adverse reactions are recorded at 15-minute intervals.

About Written Drug Orders

_____ 1. Should include the patient's name.

_____ 2. Should include the name of the drug to be administered.

_____ 3. Should include who is to administer the drug.

_____ 4. Should include what dosage route and form of the drug are to be used.

_____ 5. Should include the dose to be administered.

_____ 6. Should include the frequency of administration.

About Guidelines for Preparing a Drug for Administration

_____ 1. The written orders should be checked.

_____ 2. The drug label should be checked only once.

_____ 3. Never remove a drug from an unlabeled container.

_____ 4. Deposit capsules and tablets into clean hands then drop into medicine cup.

_____ 5. Replace the caps of drug containers immediately after the drug is removed.

_____ 6. Return drugs requiring special storage immediately to their storage area.

_____ 7. Follow aseptic technique when handling syringes and needles.

About Patient Care Considerations for Oral Drug Administration

_____ 1. A full glass of water should be given.

_____ 2. The patient may take the oral drug in any position.

_____ 3. The healthcare provider may safely leave the drug for the patient to take when convenient.

_____ 4. Patients with nasogastric feeding tubes may have their medication given through the tube.

_____ 5. Sublingual drugs must not be chewed or swallowed.

About Patient Care Considerations for Parenteral Drug Administration

_____ 1. Gloves must be worn for protection from a potential blood spill.

_____ 2. Cleanse the skin at the site of injection.

_____ 3. After insertion of the needle for an IM injection, blood should appear in the syringe after pulling back on the barrel.

_____ 4. After insertion of the needle for an IV drug administration, blood should appear in the syringe after pulling back on the barrel.

_____ 5. Syringes are not recapped but are disposed of according to policy.

_____ 6. There is no need to place pressure on an injection site from an IV, SC, or IM injection.

V. FILL IN THE BLANK

Fill in the blanks using words from the list below.

11	15
circular	standing
outward	skin
inner	muscle
administration	surgical
45	topical
inhalation	90
immediately	

1. When a drug error occurs it must be reported _____ .

2. Most drug errors are made during _____ .

3. A _____ order is one that is written when the patient is to receive the prescribed drug on a regular basis.

4. The skin site for parenteral drug administration is cleansed using a(n) _____ motion from a(n) _____ point and moving _____ .

5. A Sharps Inquiry Log must be kept by employers with _____ or more employees.

6. A subcutaneous injection places the drug into the tissues between the _____ and the _____ .

7. In an SC injection, the needle is placed at a _____ degree angle, in an IM injection the needle is inserted at a _____ degree angle, and in an intradermal injection the needle is placed at a _____ degree angle.

8. A venous access port requires _____ implantation and removal.

9. Drugs that are used to soften, disinfect, or lubricate the skin are _____ drugs.

10. Examples of drugs administered by _____ include mucolytics, anti-inflammatories, and bronchodilators.

VI. LIST

List the requested number of items.

1. List the six rights of drug administration.

   a. _____

   b. _____

   c. _____

   d. _____

   e. _____

   f. _____

2. List the three times that a drug label should be checked.

   a. _____

   b. _____

   c. _____

3. List the three forms of oral drugs.

   a. _____

   b. _____

   c. _____

4. List the four most commonly used routes of administration of parenteral drugs.

   a. _____

   b. _____

   c. _____

   d. _____

5. List six diseases that can be transmitted by needle exposures or sticks.

   a. _____

   b. _____

   c. _____

   d. _____

   e. _____

   f. _____

6. List three sites for SC injections.

    a. _____

    b. _____

    c. _____

7. List four parenteral routes of drug administration that may be done by a healthcare provider.

    a. _____

    b. _____

    c. _____

    d. _____

8. List five items that should be known by the healthcare professional involved in the administration of drugs.

    a. _____

    b. _____

    c. _____

    d. _____

    e. _____

9. List four precautions that should be followed to prevent drug errors before administration.

    a. _____

    b. _____

    c. _____

    d. _____

VII. CLINICAL APPLICATION

1. Mr. T is being discharged from the hospital but will need to continue his medications at home. As a healthcare professional, what might you ask or suggest to Mr. T regarding his home environment and safe drug administration?

2. Today is the first day of employment for Miss C in a clinical setting of more than 20 persons. What OSHA guidelines should she be informed of before she begins using needles?

3 Patient and Family Teaching

I. MATCHING

Match the term from Column A with the correct definition from Column B.

COLUMN A

_____ 1. affective domain

_____ 2. cognitive domain

_____ 3. learning

_____ 4. motivation

_____ 5. teaching

COLUMN B

A. The desire for, or seeing the need for, something.
B. An interactive process that promotes learning.
C. Acquiring new knowledge of skills.
D. Refers to one's attitudes, feelings, beliefs, and opinions.
E. Refers to intellectual activities such as thought, recall, decision making, and drawing conclusions.

II. TRUE/FALSE

Indicate whether each statement is True (T) or False (F).

_____ 1. Learning can occur in two of the three domains.

_____ 2. The affective domain of a patient can be learned about by encouraging the patient to express his or her thoughts and feelings.

_____ 3. Adults learn only what they feel they need to learn.

_____ 4. All patients learning about the same medication need the same information.

_____ 5. All drugs can potentially cause adverse reactions.

_____ 6. Patients learn best about their drugs immediately before discharge.

_____ 7. Repetition usually enhances learning.

III. MULTIPLE CHOICE

Circle the letter of the best answer.

1. Healthcare instructors consider a patient's cognitive abilities when they give him or her information about _____.
   a. adverse reactions that may occur
   b. his or her medication regimen
   c. his or her disease process
   d. answers a and b are correct
   e. answers a, b, and c are correct

2. Teaching a patient to inject insulin or take oral medications properly is an example of learning in the _____.
   a. cognitive domain
   b. psychomotor domain
   c. affective domain
   d. answers a and c are correct
   e. answers a, b, and c are correct

3. To teach a patient about medication, the healthcare instructor should _____.
   a. identify the patient's knowledge and skills
   b. devise a plan of care to meet the patient's needs
   c. do the teaching
   d. evaluate the effectiveness of the teaching
   e. all of the answers are correct

4. To determine the patient's learning needs, the healthcare instructor must evaluate what the patient needs to learn by assessing the _____.
   a. barriers or obstacles to learning that the patient faces
   b. patient's ability to learn, accept, and use the information
   c. information the patient needs to know about the drug
   d. answers a and b are correct
   e. all of the answers are correct

5. A typical teaching plan for patient education includes information on all of the following except _____.
   a. drug containers and storage of drugs
   b. dosage regimen

c. possible adverse reactions
d. basic information about drugs
e. role of family members

6. An individual patient's ability to learn can be assessed by evaluating all the following except _____.
   a. if the patient has a learning impairment
   b. if the patient is left-handed or right-handed
   c. if the patient has difficulty reading
   d. if the patient has difficulty communicating
   e. the educational level of the patient

IV. RECALL FACTS

Indicate which of the following statements are Facts with an F. If the statement is not a fact, leave the line blank.

About Dosage Regimens

_____ 1. A patient should never increase or decrease the dosage of a drug unless directed by the healthcare provider.

_____ 2. A prescribed drug may be stopped whenever the patient feels ready to end the medication.

_____ 3. The advantage of capsules is that they may be chewed or swallowed whole based on the patient's ability to swallow.

_____ 4. Capsules or tablets should be taken with a full glass of water unless directed otherwise by the healthcare provider.

_____ 5. The patient should keep a list of the exact names of all drugs, both prescription and nonprescription, currently being taken in their wallets or purse for reference.

_____ 6. The patient should not double the next dose of a drug if it is omitted or forgotten.

About Drugs, Drug Containers, and Drug Storage

_____ 1. The term "drug" applies to both prescription and nonprescription drugs.

_____ 2. It is not a problem to place two or more different drugs in one container; in fact, it makes it easier for the patient.

_____ 3. All directions printed on the label of a drug must be followed to ensure effectiveness.

_____ 4. Drugs may be stored anywhere that is convenient for the patient, regardless of what the label states.

_____ 5. If a drug changes color or develops a new odor, the pharmacist should be consulted.

_____ 6. It is permissible for elderly patients to put their drugs in other containers that are easier to open.

V. FILL IN THE BLANK

Fill in the blanks using words from the list below.

teaching process	a day or more
should not	motivation
domain	affective
two or more	

1. Hospitalized patients _____ be taught in the presence of non-family visitors.

2. Teaching of hospitalized patients should be started _____ before discharge.

3. Material may need to be presented to the patient in _____ sessions for effective learning to occur.

4. A patient must have _____ to learn.

5. The _____ is the means through which the patient is made aware of the drug regimen.

6. A _____ is a set of related human characteristics and skills.

7. The best way to learn about a patient's _____ behavior is to develop a therapeutic relationship based on trust and caring.

VI. LIST

List the requested number of items.

1. List three points about adverse reactions that should be included in a teaching plan.
   a. _____
   b. _____
   c. _____

2. List two points about family members that should be included in a teaching plan.

    a. _____

    b. _____

VII. CLINICAL APPLICATIONS

1. Mrs. W is being discharged from the hospital and will need to continue her prescribed drug therapy for several more weeks. She is elderly and lives alone. Her drug therapy involves multi-ple drugs taken at different times during the day and evening. Her daughter says that she will stop by once a day to be sure that her mother is taking her medications at the prescribed time. What can you do or suggest to help Miss W with her home drug administration regimen?

2. Your neighbor, who has difficulty with English, has been ill. After returning home from her doctor's appointment, she brings you all the non-prescription medications she has been told to take for her disorder. Since you speak her native language, what do you think would be helpful for her to know about her medications?

4 Drugs That Affect the Neurological System

I. MATCHING

Match the term from Column A with the correct definition from Column B.

COLUMN A

_____ 1. cardiac arrhythmia

_____ 2. cholinergic crisis

_____ 3. first dose effect

_____ 4. neurotransmitter

_____ 5. orthostatic hypotension

_____ 6. postural hypotension

_____ 7. shock

_____ 8. vasopressor

_____ 9. peripheral nervous system

_____ 10. autonomic nervous system

COLUMN B

A. A life-threatening condition occurring when the supply of arterial blood flow and oxygen to the cells and tissues is inadequate.

B. The branch of the peripheral nervous system that controls functions essential for survival.

C. Irregular heartbeat.

D. A drug that raises the blood pressure because it constricts blood vessels.

E. A feeling of light-headedness and dizziness after suddenly changing from a lying to a sitting or standing position.

F. A feeling of light-headedness and dizziness after suddenly changing position after standing in one place for a long period.

G. All nerves outside the brain and spinal cord, connecting all parts of the body with the central nervous system.

H. Cholinergic drug toxicity.

I. A chemical substance released at nerve ending to help transmit nerve impulses.

J. An unusually strong therapeutic effect experienced by some patients with the first dose of a medication.

II. MATCHING

Match the item in Column A with the correct definition from Column B.

COLUMN A

_____ 1. central nervous system (CNS)

_____ 2. peripheral nervous system (PNS)

_____ 3. somatic nervous system (SNS)

_____ 4. autonomic nervous system (ANS)

_____ 5. parasympathetic nervous system

_____ 6. sympathetic nervous system

COLUMN B

A. The branch of the PNS that controls functions essential for life.

B. The branch of the PNS that controls sensation and voluntary movement.

C. The branch of the ANS that regulates the expenditure of body energy.

D. Consists of the brain and spinal cord.

E. All nerves outside the brain and spinal cord.

F. The branch of the ANS that helps to conserve body energy.

III. MATCHING

Match the generic adrenergic or adrenergic blocking drug in Column A with the trade name of the drug in Column B.

COLUMN A

_____ 1. phentolamine

_____ 2. dopamine

_____ 3. isoproterenol

_____ 4. midodrine

_____ 5. betaxolol

_____ 6. dobutamine HCl

_____ 7. metoprolol

_____ 8. propranolol

_____ 9. levalbuterol

_____ 10. labetalol

_____ 11. clonidine HCl

_____ 12. metaraminol

COLUMN B

A. Xopenex
B. ProAmatine
C. Dobutrex
D. Regitine
E. Intropin
F. Isuprel
G. Aramine
H. Kerlone
I. Normodyne
J. Catapres
K. Lopressor

IV. MATCHING

Match the adrenergic drug or adrenergic blocking drug in Column A with the corresponding contraindication from Column B.

COLUMN A

_____ 1. isoproterenol

_____ 2. alpha-adrenergic blocking drugs

_____ 3. dopamine

_____ 4. beta-adrenergic blocking drugs

_____ 5. epinephrine

_____ 6. norepinephrine

_____ 7. antiadrenergic blocking drugs (centrally acting)

_____ 8. antiadrenergic blocking drugs (peripherally acting)

_____ 9. midodrine

COLUMN B

A. Narrow angle glaucoma
B. Severe organic heart disease
C. Pheochromocytoma
D. Sinus bradycardia, asthma
E. Active hepatic disease
F. Coronary artery disease
G. Pregnancy and lactation
H. Tachyarrhythmias
I. Hypotension caused by blood loss

V. MATCHING

Match the generic cholinergic or cholinergic blocking drug in Column A with the corresponding trade name from Column B.

COLUMN A

_____ 1. ambenonium

_____ 2. flavoxate

_____ 3. tridihexethyl chloride

_____ 4. glycopyrrolate

_____ 5. pyridostigmine bromide

_____ 6. bethanechol chloride

_____ 7. clidinium bromide

_____ 8. methscopolamine

_____ 9. neostigmine

_____ 10. pilocarpine HCl

COLUMN B

A. Duvoid, Urecholine
B. Isopto Carpine, Pilocar
C. Urispas
D. Pamine
E. Mytelase
F. Mestinon
G. Prostigmin
H. Robinul
I. Pathilon
J. Quarzan

VI. TRUE/FALSE

Indicate whether each statement is True (T) or False (F).

_____ 1. Adrenergic nerve fibers have only alpha- or beta-receptors.

_____ 2. Adrenergic drugs may bind to alpha-, beta-, or alpha-/beta-receptor sites.

_____ 3. Beta-adrenergic blocking drugs work to stimulate receptors in the heart and cause the heart rate to increase.

_____ 4. Beta-adrenergic blocking drugs can result in a greater risk of adverse reactions for older adults.

_____ 5. Centrally acting anti-adrenergic drugs have a different action than peripherally acting anti-adrenergic drugs, but both produce the same basic results.

_____ 6. Adverse reactions of peripherally acting anti-adrenergic drugs include dry mouth, drowsiness, anorexia, and weakness.

_____ 7. Peripheral vasodilation is the result of administering an alpha-/beta-adrenergic blocking drug.

_____ 8. A direct-acting cholinergic drug acts like the neurohormone acetylcholine.

_____ 9. Cholinergic drugs, with the exception of topical administration, are selective and specific receptor-dependent in their actions.

_____ 10. Cholinergic blocking drugs have a variety of uses because of their widespread effects on many organs and structures.

VII. MULTIPLE CHOICE

Circle the letter of the best answer.

1. _____ mimic the activity of the sympathetic nervous system.
   a. Cholinergic drugs
   b. Adrenergic drugs
   c. Cholinergic blocking drugs
   d. Adrenergic blocking drugs
   e. None of the answers are correct

2. _____ block the action of the neurotransmitter acetylcholine in the parasympathetic nervous system.
   a. Cholinergic drugs
   b. Adrenergic drugs
   c. Adrenergic blocking drugs
   d. Cholinergic blocking drugs
   e. None of the answers are correct

3. Adrenergic drugs generally produce which of the following responses?
   a. increased heart rate
   b. increased use of glucose
   c. wakefulness
   d. relaxation of smooth muscles of the bronchi
   e. all of the answers are correct

4. Adrenergic drugs can be used to treat shock because they _____ .
   a. decrease cardiac output and cause vasodilation
   b. improve myocardial contractility and cause vasoconstriction
   c. allow hypotension to occur
   d. cause bradycardia
   e. can keep the kidneys, brain, and heart alive

5. All of the following, except one, is a common adverse reaction of adrenergic drugs. Indicate the exception.
   a. cardiac arrhythmias
   b. headache
   c. insomnia
   d. drowsiness
   e. increased blood pressure

6. Alpha-adrenergic blocking drugs _____ .
   a. stimulate vasodilation
   b. can be used to treat hypertension from pheochromocytoma
   c. may have adverse reactions of weakness, orthostatic hypotension, or cardiac arrhythmias
   d. are contraindicated in patients with coronary artery disease
   e. all of the answers are correct

7. In which of the following conditions are beta-adrenergic blocking drugs used for treatment?
   a. hypertension
   b. congestive heart failure
   c. glaucoma
   d. cardiac arrhythmias
   e. answers a, c, and d are correct

8. Patients in whom beta-adrenergic drugs are contraindicated are those _____ .
   a. with a known hypersensitivity to the drugs
   b. with sinus bradycardia
   c. with heart failure
   d. with asthma or emphysema
   e. all of the answers are correct

9. Antiadrenergic drugs are used mainly for the treatment of _____ .
   a. myocardial infarction
   b. narrow angle glaucoma
   c. gastrointestinal disorders
   d. cardiac arrhythmias and hypertension
   e. active liver disease

10. Which patient should not be prescribed an alpha-/beta-adrenergic blocking drug?
    a. a patient with diarrhea
    b. a patient with bronchial asthma
    c. a patient with myocardial infarction
    d. a patient with a gastrointestinal disorder
    e. a patient with hypotension

11. Cholinergic drugs are commonly used to treat patients with _____ .
    a. myocardial infarction
    b. glaucoma
    c. myasthenia gravis
    d. urinary retention
    e. answers b, c, and d are correct

12. Which of the following cholinergic drugs might be prescribed for a patient with myasthenia gravis?
    a. pilocarpine
    b. ambenonium
    c. pyridostigmine
    d. bethanechol chloride
    e. either answer b or c

13. Cholinergic blocking drugs, such as pilocarpine HCl, work by _____ .
    a. stimulating acetylcholinesterase production
    b. inhibiting the activity of acetylcholine in parasympathetic nerve fibers
    c. stimulating sympathetic nerve fibers in selected areas of the body
    d. allowing the patient to specifically control one organ system
    e. none of the answers are correct

14. A patient in a cholinergic crisis may exhibit all *except* which of the following symptoms?
    a. severe abdominal cramping
    b. clenching of the jaw
    c. migraine headache
    d. excessive salivation
    e. diarrhea

15. A patient receiving a cholinergic drug for treatment of myasthenia gravis _____ .
    a. may require the drug every 2 to 4 hours
    b. must be observed for symptoms of drug overdose
    c. must be observed for symptoms of drug underdose
    d. may be able to use sustained release tablets
    e. all of the answers are correct

16. Ephedra is _____ .
    a. an amphetamine-like compound with stimulant effects
    b. considered safe for all patients
    c. can produce serious side effects including stroke and death
    d. approved for use by all athletic organizations
    e. answers a and c are correct

VIII. RECALL FACTS

Indicate which of the following statements are Facts with an F. If the statement is not a fact, leave the line blank.

About Managing Adverse Reactions of Cholinergic Blocking Agents

_____ 1. Heat prostration may be a problem for elderly or debilitated patients in hot weather.

_____ 2. Elderly patients receiving a cholinergic blocking drug should be observed closely for signs of mental confusion, agitation, or other adverse reactions.

_____ 3. Photophobia and blurred vision is rarely a concern for patients on cholinergic blocking agents.

_____ 4. Mouth dryness will go away after the drug is used for awhile.

_____ 5. Objects that may obstruct walking should be moved out of the patients' way.

_____ 6. Patients experiencing constipation, who are not fluid restricted, may increase their fluid intake up to 2000 ml per day.

Indicate whether the listed adrenergic blocking drug is an alpha (A), a beta (B), or an alpha/beta (AB) drug.

About Adrenergic Blocking Drugs

_____ 1. carvedilol

_____ 2. acebutolol

_____ 3. phentolamine

_____ 4. metoprolol

_____ 5. propanolol

_____ 6. labetalol

IX. FILL IN THE BLANK

Fill in the blanks using words from the list below.

5–10 minutes   glaucoma
cholinergic blocking drug   atropine
first dose effect   midodrine
congestive heart failure

1. Supine hypertension is a potentially dangerous adverse reaction of _____ .

2. A serious adverse reaction of beta-adrenergic blocking drugs includes symptoms of _____ .

3. A(n) _____ is generally self-limiting and in most cases does not recur after the initial period of therapy.

4. The anti-cholinergic drug, _____, is used as an antidote to cholinergic drug over-dose.

5. A common adverse reaction of a(n) _____ is dryness of the mouth.

6. Cholinergic blocking drugs are contraindicated in patients with _____ .

7. A patient being treated with a cholinergic drug for urinary retention can expect urination to occur within _____ of subcutaneous drug administration.

X. LIST

List the requested number of items.

1. List four conditions that adrenergic drugs may be used to treat.

   a. _____

   b. _____

   c. _____

   d. _____

2. List the five types of shock.

   a. _____

   b. _____

   c. _____

   d. _____

   e. _____

3. List the four groups of adrenergic blocking drugs with the effects on the body.

	Group	Effect
a.	_____	_____
b.	_____	_____
c.	_____	_____
d.	_____	_____

4. List four examples of beta-adrenergic blocking drugs.

   a. _____

   b. _____

   c. _____

   d. _____

5. List four things that a healthcare worker could do to help a patient minimize the adverse reaction of hypotension.

   a. _____

   b. _____

   c. _____

   d. _____

6. List three drugs that can be used to treat myasthenia gravis.

   a. _____

   b. _____

   c. _____

XI. CLINICAL APPLICATIONS

1. Mrs. P's healthcare provider has prescribed Banthine, a cholinergic blocking drug for the treatment of her neurogenic bladder. Knowing that a dry mouth is a common adverse reaction of this medication, the healthcare provider asks you to give Mrs. P some helpful hints for dealing with the potential problem. What might you suggest to Mrs. P to help her?

2. Your father has been diagnosed with hypertension and must monitor his blood pressure daily at home. What could you suggest to your father to help ensure that he gets an accurate blood pressure reading?

I. MATCHING

Match the term from Column A with the correct definition from Column B.

COLUMN A

_____ 1. ataxia

_____ 2. bipolar disorder

_____ 3. dysphoric

_____ 4. dystonia

_____ 5. endogenous

_____ 6. photophobia

_____ 7. psychotic disorder

_____ 8. soporific

_____ 9. tardive dyskinesia

_____ 10. tolerance

COLUMN B

A. Extreme or exaggerated sadness, anxiety, or unhappiness.

B. A psychiatric disorder characterized by severe mood swings from extreme hyperactivity to depression.

C. Made within the body.

D. Another term for a hypnotic drug.

E. Facial grimacing and twisting of the neck into unnatural positions.

F. Unsteady gait.

G. A disorder characterized by extreme personality disorganization and a loss of contact with reality.

H. An intolerance to light.

I. A syndrome consisting of potentially irreversible, involuntary dyskinetic movements.

J. Patient condition in which increasingly larger dosages are required to obtain the desired effect.

II. MATCHING

Match the generic name of the sedative or hypnotic from Column A with the correct trade name from Column B.

COLUMN A

_____ 1. amobarbital sodium

_____ 2. zaleplon

_____ 3. phenobarbital

_____ 4. zolpidem tartrate

_____ 5. pentobarbital sodium

_____ 6. ethchlorvynol

_____ 7. flurazepam

_____ 8. temazepam

_____ 9. aprobarbital

_____ 10. mephobarbital

COLUMN B

A. Luminal, Bellatal
B. Placidyl
C. Sonata
D. Amytal sodium
E. Ambien
F. Dalmane
G. Restoril
H. Nembutal sodium
I. Alurate
J. Mebaral

III. MATCHING

Match the antidepressant drug from Column A with the action from Column B.

COLUMN A

_____ 1. MAOIs

_____ 2. TCAs

_____ 3. SSRIs

_____ 4. Miscellaneous antidepressants

COLUMN B

A. Inhibit uptake of norepinephrine or serotonin at the presynaptic neuron.
B. Not understood.
C. Inhibit the uptake of serotonin.
D. Inhibit the activity of monoamine oxidase.

IV. MATCHING

Match the generic antipsychotic drug from Column A with the correct trade name from Column B.

COLUMN A

_____ 1. ziprasidone

_____ 2. risperidone

_____ 3. prochlorperazine

_____ 4. chlorpromazine

_____ 5. haloperidol

_____ 6. pimozide

_____ 7. lithium

_____ 8. olanzapine

_____ 9. perphenazine

_____ 10. quetiapine fumarate

COLUMN B

A. Compazine
B. Haldol
C. Eskalith
D. Thorazine
E. Orap
F. Risperdal
G. Seroquel
H. Geodon
I. Trilafon
J. Zyprexa

V. MATCHING

Indicate whether the drug listed in Column A is a sedative/hypnotic or an antidepressant from Column B.

COLUMN A

_____ 1. alprazolam

_____ 2. flurazepam

_____ 3. triazolam

_____ 4. diazepam

_____ 5. chlordiazepoxide

_____ 6. lorazepam

_____ 7. buspirone

_____ 8. pentobarbital sodium

_____ 9. zolpidem

_____ 10. phenobarbital

COLUMN B

A. Sedative/hypnotic
B. Antidepressant

VI. TRUE/FALSE

Indicate whether each statement is True (T) or False (F).

_____ 1. Benzodiazepines are thought to have their tranquilizing action by potentiating the effects of gamma amino butyric acid.

_____ 2. The benzodiazepines and the nonbenzodiazepines have similar actions at the cellular level.

_____ 3. Antianxiety drugs must never be discontinued abruptly because severe withdrawal symptoms may occur.

_____ 4. If depressive symptoms occur daily or nearly every day for 2 weeks or more, the episode is considered to be major.

_____ 5. Research indicates that antidepressants work by changing the brain's receptors for norepinephrine and serotonin.

_____ 6. Tricyclics are the drug of choice for treating depression in patients with preexisting cardiac disease or prostatic enlargement.

_____ 7. Sedatives and hypnotics are controlled substances.

_____ 8. Supportive care is the main treatment of barbiturate toxicity.

_____ 9. Barbiturates are often administered for their strong analgesic action.

_____ 10. Patients should not drink alcohol while taking sedatives or hypnotics because there is an additive effect which increases the central nervous system depression.

_____ 11. Benzodiazepines are also called antianxiety drugs.

_____ 12. Sedatives and hypnotics are generally divided into two classes: the barbiturates and miscellaneous sedatives and hypnotics.

_____ 13. The effects of sedatives or hypnotics usually diminish after approximately 2 weeks.

_____ 14. The use of barbiturates for longer than 2 weeks poses no physical or psychological dependence.

_____ 15. MAOIs are not widely used because of potential serious adverse reactions.

_____ 16. It is safe to use a miscellaneous antidepressant during pregnancy.

_____ 17. St. John's wort is useful for treating mild to moderate depression.

_____ 18. Reducing the dosage of the antipsychotic drug will usually reduce extrapyramidal effects.

_____ 19. Patients taking lithium should lower their fluid intake to keep a higher concentration of the drug in their system for a longer period.

_____ 20. Frequent assessments are necessary for patients taking antipsychotics over the long term, because dosage adjustments may be necessary.

VII. MULTIPLE CHOICE

Circle the letter of the best answer.

1. Which of the following is not a group of barbiturates?
   a. ultra-short-acting
   b. short-acting
   c. intermediate acting
   d. long-acting
   e. ultra-long-acting

2. Barbiturates generally act by _____ .
   a. depressing the central nervous system
   b. causing mood alteration
   c. causing respiratory depression
   d. answers a and b are correct
   e. answers a, b, and c are correct

3. Sedatives and hypnotics may be used _____ .
   a. to treat anxiety
   b. to treat insomnia
   c. as part of a preoperative regimen
   d. to help manage an illness
   e. all of the answers are correct

4. Patient's respiratory function should be monitored _____ sedative or hypnotic use.
   a. before
   b. 30 minutes to 1 hour after
   c. frequently after 1 hour
   d. answers a and c are correct
   e. answers a, b, and c are correct

5. Valerian works to treat insomnia by _____ .
   a. relaxing muscles
   b. reducing awakenings
   c. shortening the time it takes to fall asleep
   d. answers a and b are correct
   e. answers a, b, and c are correct

6. Common adverse reactions with SSRIs include all of the following except _____ .
   a. headache
   b. nervousness
   c. insomnia
   d. congestive heart failure
   e. nausea

7. Adverse reactions of bupropion include insomnia, but Trazodone may cause _____ .
   a. drowsiness
   b. headache
   c. dry mouth
   d. constipation
   e. seizures

8. St. John's wort has been used to treat _____ .
   a. insect bites
   b. wounds and burns
   c. depression
   d. sleep disorders
   e. all of the answers are correct

9. Antipsychotic drugs are thought to act by _____ .
   a. blocking the release of dopamine in the brain
   b. increasing the firing of neurons in areas of the brain
   c. inhibiting MAO
   d. stimulating the release of dopamine in the brain
   e. answers a and b are correct

10. Chlorpromazine can be used _____ .
    a. as an antipsychotic
    b. as an antiemetic

c. to treat uncontrollable hiccoughs
d. answers a and c are correct
e. answers a, b, and c are correct

11. All of the following are extrapyramidal effects except _____ .
    a. akathisia
    b. Parkinson-like symptoms
    c. dystonia
    d. paranoid reactions
    e. none of the answers are correct

12. Tardive dyskinesia _____ .
    a. has potentially irreversible involuntary dyskinetic movements
    b. has no known treatment
    c. has a higher incidence in older women
    d. symptoms signal that the drug must be discontinued
    e. all of the answers are correct

13. Oral liquid concentrates are _____ .
    a. light sensitive
    b. the cause of gastrointestinal adverse effects
    c. available in many flavors
    d. administered mixed in liquids such as juices and carbonated beverages
    e. answers a and d are correct

14. Two types of antianxiety drugs are _____ .
    a. sedatives and hypnotics
    b. barbiturates and nonbarbiturates
    c. MAOIs and COMTs
    d. benzodiazepines and nonbenzodiazepines
    e. none of the answers are correct

15. Which of the following antianxiety drugs is not a benzodiazepine?
    a. alprazolam
    b. hydroxyzine
    c. diazepam
    d. lorazepam
    e. chlordiazepoxide

16. Antianxiety drugs _____ .
    a. are not recommended for long-term therapy
    b. can result in drug dependence
    c. can also be used as sedatives
    d. generally do not cause severe adverse reactions
    e. all of the answers are correct

17. An elderly patient who is experiencing anxiety might be given _____ since it does not cause excessive sedation.

    a. buspirone
    b. clorazepate
    c. diazepam
    d. lorazepam
    e. oxazepam

18. When benzodiazepine toxicity occurs, which of the following drugs can be given as an antidote?
    a. nonbenzodiazepines
    b. flurazepam
    c. flumazenil
    d. lithium
    e. GABA

19. Other than in patients with a known hypersensitivity, in which conditions are antianxiety drugs contraindicated?
    a. shock or coma
    b. narrow angle glaucoma
    c. pregnancy and labor
    d. acute alcoholic intoxication
    e. all of the answers are correct

20. In which of the following conditions are TCAs contraindicated?
    a. recent myocardial infarction
    b. pregnancy and lactation
    c. patients about to receive or having just had a myelogram
    d. within 14 days of using an MAOI
    e. all of the answers are correct

VIII. RECALL FACTS

Indicate which of the following statements are Facts with an F. If the statement is not a fact, leave the line blank.

About Adverse Reactions of Sedative and Hypnotics

_____ 1. The patient must be protected from harm with a safe environment when experiencing excitement or confusion.

_____ 2. No additional doses of hypnotics may be given if a patient awakens during the night.

_____ 3. If a patient experiences a drug hangover, the healthcare provider should be notified.

_____ 4. Elderly patients are at a greater risk for oversedation, dizziness, and confusion.

About Patient Management Issues with Antianxiety Drugs

_____ 1. Anxious patients generally have cool, pale skin.

_____ 2. Only hospitalized patients may receive nonbenzodiazepines.

_____ 3. Prolonged therapy may lead to dependence.

_____ 4. Parenteral administration is the safest way for elderly or debilitated patients to receive antianxiety drugs.

About Kava

_____ 1. Kava is a popular treatment for reducing stress, anxiety, and depression.

_____ 2. Kava is safe to use on a long-term basis.

_____ 3. The FDA has issued an alert that the use of kava may cause liver damage.

_____ 4. Kava is also known as ava, kew, sakau, tonga, or yangona.

_____ 5. Kavaism indicates that the herb is working.

About Contraindications, Precautions, and Interactions of Antipsychotic Drugs

_____ 1. Antipsychotics are contraindicated in pregnant or lactating women.

_____ 2. Patients who have a hypersensitivity to tartrazine should not take lithium.

_____ 3. Taking an antipsychotic drug with alcohol may result in additive CNS depression.

_____ 4. Antipsychotics are used commonly in patients exposed to extreme heat or phosphorus insecticides.

_____ 5. Clozapine works synergistically with other drugs that suppress bone marrow.

IX. FILL IN THE BLANK

Fill in the blanks using words from the list below.

drug dependency	anxiolytic drug
insomnia	tyramine
haloperidol	fatal reaction
St. John's wort	lithium
Kava	MAOIs

1. A(n) _____ is used to treat anxiety.

2. _____ is classified as a dietary supplement.

3. Orthostatic hypertension is not a common adverse reaction of _____ .

4. Food containing _____ can cause a serious hypertensive crisis when eaten by a patient taking an MAOI.

5. Melatonin's most significant use is for the short-term treatment of _____ .

6. If sertraline is taken with an MAOI, a potentially _____ can occur.

7. Patients may not safely use _____ in conjunction with any other antidepressant.

8. _____ is an antimanic drug which seems to alter sodium transport in nerve and muscle cells.

9. Neuroleptic malignant syndrome, which is an adverse reaction of antipsychotic drugs, most often occurs in patients taking _____ .

10. Sedatives and hypnotics are generally not given for longer than 2 weeks because of potential _____ .

X. LIST

List the requested number of items.

1. List the three types of psychotherapeutic drugs used to treat mental illness.

   a. _____

   b. _____

   c. _____

2. List four adverse reactions associated with the use of barbiturates as a sedative or hypnotic.

   a. _____

   b. _____

c. _____

d. _____

3. List four types of patients in which sedative or hypnotic administration is contraindicated.

a. _____

b. _____

c. _____

d. _____

4. List three symptoms that would indicate to the healthcare provider that a sedative or hypnotic should be withheld.

a. _____

b. _____

c. _____

5. List three facts about adverse effects of clozapine.

a. _____

b. _____

c. _____

6. List five symptoms of a major depressive episode.

a. _____

b. _____

c. _____

d. _____

e. _____

7. List the two most common adverse reactions of TCAs.

a. _____

b. _____

8. List four conditions in which the use of MAOIs is contraindicated.

a. _____

b. _____

c. _____

d. _____

9. List three drugs used to treat schizophrenia.

a. _____

b. _____

c. _____

10. List three important adverse reactions of anti-psychotics.

a. _____

b. _____

c. _____

XI. CLINICAL APPLICATION

1. Miss K has decided on her own that after 6 weeks of treatment with a barbiturate that she no longer needs to take the medication. What are some of the symptoms that Miss K may experience as she goes through withdrawal of the drug?

2. The healthcare provider has asked you to explain to Mr. G some general information about taking his antidepressant medication. What key things should Mr. G know about using these drugs?

Central Nervous System Stimulants, Anticonvulsants, and Antiparkinsonism Drugs

I. MATCHING

Match the term from Column A with the correct definition from Column B.

COLUMN A

_____ 1. analeptics

_____ 2. choreiform movements

_____ 3. dystonic movements

_____ 4. epilepsy

_____ 5. Jacksonian seizure

_____ 6. narcolepsy

_____ 7. pancytopenia

_____ 8. psychomotor seizures

_____ 9. status epilepticus

_____ 10. tonic-clonic seizures

COLUMN B

A. An emergency situation characterized by continual seizure activity with no interruptions.
B. A decrease in all the cellular components of the blood.
C. A focal seizure that begins with uncontrolled stiffening or jerking of a part of the body, such as the finger, mouth, hand, or foot, that may progress to a generalized seizure.
D. A permanent, recurrent seizure disorder.
E. Drugs that stimulate the respiratory center.
F. An alternate contraction and relaxation of muscles, a loss of consciousness, and abnormal behavior.
G. The involuntary twitching of the limbs or facial muscles.
H. A disorder causing an uncontrollable desire to sleep during normal waking hours.
I. A seizure that may involve an aura with perceptual alterations, such as hallucinations or a strong sense of fear; most often occurs in children through adolescence.
J. Muscular spasms most often affecting the tongue, jaw, eyes, and neck.

II. MATCHING

Match the generic CNS stimulant drug in Column A with the trade name of the drug in Column B.

COLUMN A

_____ 1. dextroamphetamine

_____ 2. pemoline

_____ 3. caffeine

_____ 4. modafinil

_____ 5. doxapram HCl

_____ 6. methamphetamine

_____ 7. dexmethylphenidate

_____ 8. methylphenidate HCl

_____ 9. diethylpropion HCl

_____ 10. phentermine HCl

_____ 11. sibutramine HCl

_____ 12. benzphetamine HCl

COLUMN B

A. Desoxyn
B. Provigil
C. Dopram
D. Focalin
E. Dexedrine
F. Caffedrine
G. Concerta
H. Cylert
I. Didrex
J. Ionamin
K. Meridia
L. Tenuate

III. MATCHING

Match the CNS stimulant or anticonvulsant generic drug in Column A with the drug use in Column B.

COLUMN A

_____ 1. caffeine

_____ 2. phenobarbital sodium

_____ 3. doxapram HCl

_____ 4. amphetamine sulfate

_____ 5. clorazepate

_____ 6. dexmethylphenidate

_____ 7. sibutramine HCl

_____ 8. ethotoin

_____ 9. ethosuximide

_____ 10. mephenytoin

_____ 11. oxcarbazepine

_____ 12. modafinil

_____ 13. primidone

_____ 14. methylphenidate HCl

COLUMN B

A. Drug-induced respiratory depression
B. Obesity
C. ADHD
D. Narcolepsy, ADHD, exogenous obesity
E. Narcolepsy
F. ADHD, narcolepsy
G. Status epilepticus
H. Absence seizures
 I. Tonic-clonic seizures, psychomotor seizures
 J. Partial seizures, anxiety disorders
K. Jacksonian seizures
L. Epilepsy
M. Grand mal seizures

IV. MATCHING

Match the generic antiparkinsonism drug in Column A with the trade name of the drug in Column B.

COLUMN A

_____ 1. entacapone

_____ 2. benztropine mesylate

_____ 3. amantadine

_____ 4. procyclidine

_____ 5. biperiden

_____ 6. carbidopa

_____ 7. diphenhydramine

_____ 8. levodopa

_____ 9. trihexyphenidyl

_____ 10. ropinirole HCl

_____ 11. tolcapone

_____ 12. pergolide

COLUMN B

A. Permax
B. Benadryl
C. Cogentin
D. Lodosyn
E. Akineton
F. Kemadrin
G. Symmetrel
H. Artane
 I. Requip
 J. Dopar
K. Comtan
L. Tasmar

V. TRUE/FALSE

Indicate whether each statement is True (T) or False (F).

_____ 1. Analeptics are drugs that depress the respiratory center.

_____ 2. Doxapram's action is to increase the depth of respirations by stimulating receptors located in the carotid arteries and the upper aorta.

_____ 3. Phentermine and phendimetrazine are amphetamines.

_____ 4. Phenylpropanolamine, when used as an anorexiant, has no addiction potential.

_____ 5. Amphetamines and anorexiants may be abused and can result in addiction.

_____ 6. A child with ADHD, once medicated, never has their drug regimen interrupted.

_____ 7. All seizure disorders have a known cause.

_____ 8. The on-off phenomenon that can occur in patients taking levodopa can be managed by simply abruptly stopping all medications.

_____ 9. Most anticonvulsants have specific uses and are used in the treatment of specific types of seizure disorders.

_____ 10. Anticonvulsants work by increasing the excitability of the brain, thereby reducing the intensity and frequency of neural stimulation.

_____ 11. Diazepam and phenytoin or phenobarbital are commonly given to patients experiencing status epilepticus.

_____ 12. A potentially fatal rash may occur in patients taking lamotrigine.

_____ 13. Phenytoin is contraindicated in patients with certain cardiac problems and during pregnancy and lactation.

_____ 14. Patients with bone marrow depression can be given succinimides as long as the dosage is low.

_____ 15. Antiparkinsonism drugs are used to relieve the symptoms, not cure, Parkinson's disease.

_____ 16. Oral dopamine is able to cross the blood–brain barrier and therefore is the most effective treatment for Parkinson's disease.

_____ 17. Adverse reactions with levodopa and carbidopa in the early stages of treatment are not usually a problem.

VI. MULTIPLE CHOICE

Circle the letter of the best answer.

1. Central nervous system stimulants include _____ .

   a. anticonvulsants
   b. anorexiants
   c. analeptics
   d. amphetamines
   e. answers b, c, and d are correct

2. Which of the following drugs are considered to be analeptics?

   a. modafinil
   b. caffeine
   c. doxapram
   d. phentermine
   e. answers a, b, and c are correct

3. A patient who is taking an amphetamine may have _____ .

   a. an increase in blood pressure
   b. an increase in pulse rate
   c. a decrease in pulse rate
   d. appetite suppression
   e. all of the answers except c are correct

4. All of the following except _____ are uses of amphetamines.

   a. exogenous obesity
   b. ADHD
   c. stimulation of skeletal muscle
   d. narcolepsy
   e. none of the answers are correct

5. A common adverse reaction from short-term use of amphetamines and anorexiants is _____ .

   a. drowsiness
   b. overstimulation of the CNS
   c. fever
   d. dry mouth
   e. none of the answers are correct

6. Amphetamines and anorexiants use _____ .

   a. may result in tolerance to the drug
   b. may cause psychological dependence
   c. is recommended only for short-term use for the treatment of exogenous obesity
   d. answers a and c are correct
   e. answers a, b, and c are correct

7. All of the following are true about partial seizures except _____.

   a. can cause generalized seizures
   b. arise from a localized area of the brain
   c. include simple seizures, Jacksonian seizures, and psychomotor seizures
   d. has a particular stimulus
   e. can cause specific symptoms

8. Dosages of anticonvulsants _____ .

   a. may be adjusted during times of stress or illness
   b. are often adjusted with increases or decreases during the initial period of treatment
   c. are always constant so as not to confuse the patient
   d. are only taken alone; combination therapy has not proven to be effective
   e. answers a and b are correct

9. Adverse reactions of barbiturates can include _____ .

   a. sedation
   b. agitation
   c. nausea
   d. hypersensitivity rash
   e. all of the answers are correct

10. Hydantoin's adverse reactions can include _____ .

   a. nystagmus
   b. ataxia
   c. gingival hyperplasia

d. blood dyscrasias
e. all of the answers are correct

11. Succinimides _____ .
    a. have frequent gastrointestinal symptoms
    b. rarely produce toxic effects
    c. can produce a potentially fatal rash
    d. may produce hematological changes
    e. answers a and d are correct

12. In whom should barbiturates be either contraindicated or used with precaution?
    a. hyperactive children
    b. patients with pulmonary disease
    c. patients with neurological disorders
    d. patients with a known hypersensitivity to the drug
    e. all of the answers are correct

13. Oxazolidinediones are contraindicated in patients _____.
    a. who are pregnant or lactating
    b. who have a known hypersensitivity to the drugs
    c. who have eye disorders
    d. who have liver, kidney, or neurological disorders
    e. answers a and b are correct

14. All of the following are classified as antiparkinsonism drugs except _____ .
    a. dopamine receptor agonists
    b. acetylcholinesterase inhibitors
    c. COMT inhibitors
    d. anticholinergic drugs
    e. dopaminergic drugs

15. Put the following drugs used to treat Parkinson's disease in order of most effective to least effective.
    I. carbidopa
    II. levodopa
    III. amantadine
    IV. anticholinergic
    V. dopamine
    a. I, II, III
    b. II, III, IV
    c. III, IV, V
    d. I, III, V
    e. II, IV, V

16. Choreiform and dystonic movements are the most serious and frequent adverse reactions seen with _____ .
    a. carbidopa
    b. amantadine
    c. dopamine
    d. levodopa
    e. anticholinergics

17. Adverse reactions to anticholinergic drugs commonly include dry mouth, blurred vision, dizziness, and _____ .
    a. nausea
    b. nervousness
    c. hiccoughs
    d. answers a and b
    e. all of the answers are correct

18. Patients older than 60 years of age who are taking anticholinergics _____ .
    a. require higher doses of the drugs
    b. frequently develop increased sensitivity
    c. commonly become less confused
    d. are only taking these drugs occasionally
    e. all of the answers are correct

19. COMT inhibitors are thought to act by _____ .
    a. stimulating dopamine release
    b. inhibiting acetylcholinesterase
    c. blocking an enzyme which eliminates dopamine
    d. blocking levodopa
    e. answers b and d are correct

20. Dopamine receptor agonists _____ .
    a. are thought to mimic the effects of dopamine in the brain
    b. are used to treat the signs and symptoms of Parkinson's disease
    c. have common adverse reactions of nausea, dizziness, and postural hypotension
    d. should not be given to patients with ischemic heart disease
    e. all of the answers are correct

21. Adverse reactions associated with antiparkinsonism drugs that can be managed by the healthcare provider to increase the comfort level of the patient include all the following except _____ .
    a. dry mouth
    b. urinary incontinence
    c. visual difficulties
    d. GI disturbances
    e. difficulty walking

VII. RECALL FACTS

Indicate which of the following statements are Facts with an F. If the statement is not a fact, leave the line blank.

About Managing Adverse Reactions of Anticonvulsants

_____ 1. Oral anticonvulsants are always taken on an empty stomach.

_____ 2. The patient's ability to swallow should be checked before taking any drug.

_____ 3. Precautions against injuries caused by seizures are needed until control is established.

_____ 4. Drowsiness usually decreases with continued use of the drug.

_____ 5. Barbiturates may produce excitement, depression, and confusion in older adults.

_____ 6. Diazepam is given in standard dosages to elderly patients with no difficulties.

About Patients in Whom CNS Stimulants Are Contraindicated

_____ 1. Those with a known hypersensitivity

_____ 2. Those with severe hypertension

_____ 3. Within 2 weeks of receiving an MAOI

_____ 4. Guanethidine users

_____ 5. Tricyclic antidepressant users

_____ 6. Pregnant women

_____ 7. Newborns

_____ 8. Stroke victims

_____ 9. Those with convulsive states

_____ 10. Those with glaucoma

_____ 11. Those with hyperthyroidism

_____ 12. Those with head injuries

About Patient Management Issues with Antiparkinsonism Drugs

_____ 1. Some patient histories may need to be obtained from family members.

_____ 2. The patient's neurological status needs to be established before drug therapy is started.

_____ 3. With Parkinson's disease, the healthcare provider is only concerned with monitoring drug therapy.

_____ 4. Hallucination incidence with antiparkinsonism drugs appears to increase with age.

About Managing Adverse Reactions of CNS Stimulants

_____ 1. To decrease insomnia, patients should take the drug early in the day.

_____ 2. Napping will reduce insomnia.

_____ 3. Using coffee, tea, or cola drinks will not affect the patient.

_____ 4. Increase the dosage if tolerance develops.

_____ 5. Cardiovascular disorders in elderly patients may be worsened while taking CNS stimulants; therefore. these patients should be monitored carefully.

About Anticonvulsant Management Issues

_____ 1. Anticonvulsants can cure epilepsy.

_____ 2. The dosage of an anticonvulsant is frequently adjusted during the initial treatment period.

_____ 3. Only one anticonvulsant is prescribed at a time.

_____ 4. Regular testing for drug levels is done to monitor toxicity.

_____ 5. Abrupt discontinuation of an anticonvulsant can result in status epilepticus.

_____ 6. To discontinue an anticonvulsant, gradual withdrawal of the dosage should occur.

VIII. FILL IN THE BLANK

Fill in the blanks using words from the list below.

pyridoxine	anticholinergic drugs
drowsiness	anticonvulsants
modafinil	anorexians
tolcapone	additive
insomnia	convulsion
dopamine	acetylcholine

1. _____ is believed to treat narcolepsy by increasing the alpha activity of the brain.

2. _____ generally have their action on the appetite center of the hypothalamus.

3. A common adverse reaction of the anorexiants is _____ .

4. A(n) _____ is essentially the same thing as a seizure.

5. Succinimides, oxazolidinediones, barbiturates, benzodiazepines, and hydantoins are the five types of drugs used as _____ .

6. _____ is the most common adverse reaction of oxazolidinediones.

7. The use of any of the five types of anticonvulsants with other CNS depressants can result in a(n) _____ CNS depressant effect.

8. The effect of levodopa is reversed when foods high in _____ are ingested.

9. _____ are used as adjunctive therapy in all forms of parkinsonism.

10. Liver failure is a severe and potentially fatal adverse reaction that can occur with _____ administration.

11 and 12. Parkinson's disease is a progressive, degenerative disorder of the CNS thought to be caused by a decrease in _____ and an excess of _____ .

IX. LIST

List the requested number of items.

1. List three situations in which levodopa is contraindicated.

    a. _____

    b. _____

    c. _____

2. List six drugs that interact with phenytoin.

    a. _____

    b. _____

    c. _____

    d. _____

    e. _____

    f. _____

3. List six facts about caffeine.

    a. _____

    b. _____

    c. _____

    d. _____

    e. _____

    f. _____

4. List seven types of patients in which benzodiazepines are either contraindicated or used with precaution.

    a. _____

    b. _____

    c. _____

    d. _____

    e. _____

    f. _____

    g. _____

5. List five signs of phenytoin toxicity.

    a. _____

    b. _____

    c. _____

    d. _____

    e. _____

X. CLINICAL APPLICATIONS

1. Your grandmother has been prescribed levodopa by her healthcare provider for treatment of the symptoms of her Parkinson's disease. Knowing that you are a healthcare worker, her healthcare provider asks you to make up the list of foods that your grandmother should avoid. You know that foods containing pyridoxine (vitamin B_6) may interfere with her medication, so you make up the following list of foods that your grandmother should not eat and give it to her and her home healthcare assistant.

2. A 30-year-old female co-worker has been prescribed an oxazolidinedione for her seizure disorder. The healthcare provider has asked you to go over some of the key points she should know about taking this drug.

7 Cholinesterase Inhibitors

I. MATCHING

Match the term from Column A with the correct definition from Column B.

COLUMN A

_____ 1. acetylcholine

_____ 2. Alzheimer's disease

_____ 3. alanine aminotransferase (ALT)

_____ 4. anorexia

_____ 5. dementia

_____ 6. ginkgo biloba

_____ 7. ginseng

_____ 8. hepatotoxic

COLUMN B

A. Capable of producing liver damage.
B. A diminished appetite.
C. A decrease in cognitive functioning.
D. A natural chemical in the brain that is required for memory and thinking.
E. A disease of the elderly causing progressive deterioration of mental and physical abilities.
F. An herb that appears to increase blood flow to the brain.
G. An enzyme found predominately in the liver; high levels may indicate liver damage.
H. An herb used to improve energy and mental performance.

II. MATCHING

Match the generic cholinesterase inhibitor drug from Column A with the trade name in Column B.

COLUMN A

_____ 1. galantamine hydrobromide

_____ 2. rivastigmine tartrate

_____ 3. donepezil HCl

_____ 4. tacrine HCl

COLUMN B

A. Aricept
B. Reminyl
C. Exelon, Exelon Oral Solution
D. Cognex

III. MATCHING

Match the cholinesterase inhibitor in Column A with the known drug interactions in Column B. You may use an answer more than once.

COLUMN A

_____ 1. anticholinergic drugs

_____ 2. theophylline

_____ 3. succinylcholine

_____ 4. cholinergic agonists

_____ 5. tacrine

COLUMN B

A. decrease in activity of drug
B. toxicity
C. synergistic effect

IV. TRUE OR FALSE

Indicate whether each statement is True (T) or False (F).

_____ 1. All patients respond equally well to the different cholinesterase inhibiting drugs on the market today. Therefore, it is rarely necessary to change a prescription once it is in use.

_____ 2. The adverse reactions associated with the use of cholinesterase inhibiting drugs generally last only a few days and will diminish after the body adjusts to the medication.

_____ 3. Ginkgo biloba may begin to improve symptoms after 4 to 24 weeks.

_____ 4. A patient's response to cholinesterase inhibitors is usually immediate and cures Alzheimer's disease.

_____ 5. Studies have shown that everyone using ginseng has an improvement in memory.

_____ 6. Ginkgo biloba will improve the memory of elderly patients with normal memory.

_____ 7. Ginseng use has shown only positive results in Alzheimer's patients.

_____ 8. Ginseng may interfere with digoxin.

_____ 9. Any treatment that slows the progression of symptoms in Alzheimer's disease is considered successful.

_____ 10. Ginseng is contraindicated in patients with high blood pressure and during pregnancy.

V. MULTIPLE CHOICE

Circle the letter of the best answer.

1. Acetylcholine _____ .
   a. is required for memory and thinking
   b. is slowly lost by Alzheimer's patients
   c. is a neurohormone
   d. all of the answers are correct
   e. answers a and b are correct

2. Cholinesterase inhibiting drugs _____ .
   a. act to increase the level of acetylcholine in the CNS
   b. act by inhibiting the breakdown of acetylcholine
   c. act to slow the destruction of neurons and inhibit the breakdown of acetylcholine in the brain
   d. cure Alzheimer's disease
   e. answers a, b, and c are correct

3. Cholinesterase inhibiting drugs are used to _____ .
   a. help a patient fully recover from Alzheimer's disease
   b. treat dementia associated with Alzheimer's disease
   c. replace the loss of acetylcholine in the brain
   d. accelerate the breakdown of acetylcholine and speed the destruction of neurons
   e. none of the answers are correct

4. In general, cholinesterase inhibiting drugs _____ .
   a. are effective for virtually every patient
   b. may have a variable effectiveness on an individual basis

   c. effect only males
   d. are not used on children
   e. exhibit a stimulating response

5. The drug with the fewest adverse reactions and considered to be the first drug of choice in treating Alzheimer's disease is _____ .
   a. Aricept
   b. Reminyl
   c. Exelon
   d. Cognex
   e. ALT

6. The drug _____ has the potential to be hepatotoxic and tends to cause more adverse reactions. It is also generally given in smaller and more frequent doses when it is prescribed.
   a. Aricept
   b. Reminyl
   c. Exelon
   d. Cognex
   e. ALT

7. The drug _____ appears to cause more adverse reactions such as nausea and severe vomiting.
   a. tacrine HCl
   b. galantamine hydrobromide
   c. donepezil HCl
   d. rivastigmine tartrate
   e. ginkgo biloba

8. If a patient exhibits adverse reactions _____ .
   a. the caregiver should report the reactions to the healthcare provider
   b. the healthcare provider may discontinue the medication or lower the dosage
   c. the caregiver should ignore the reaction(s), knowing they will disappear in a few days anyway
   d. the caregiver should change the dosage themselves
   e. answers a and b are correct

9. Adverse reactions such as dizziness may place a patient at risk for injury. To minimize the risk of falling, the caregiver could _____ .
   a. keep the patient in his or her room at all times
   b. restrain all patients
   c. allow the patient to roam at will
   d. provide a controlled, safe environment with assistive devices

10. A patient who is being medicated with tacrine should be monitored for _____ .
    a. liver enzyme elevations
    b. increased ALT levels

c. liver damage
d. alanine aminotransferase level elevations
e. all of the answers are correct

11. The use of cholinesterase inhibitor medication is contraindicated in which of the following patients?
    a. patients who are pregnant
    b. patients who are lactating
    c. patients with a known hypersensitivity to drugs in the cholinesterase inhibitor medication
    d. all of the above patients should not receive cholinesterase inhibitors
    e. answers b and c are correct

12. Cholinesterase inhibiting drugs may be given with caution in which of the following patients?
    a. patients with renal or hepatic disease
    b. patients with bladder obstruction
    c. patients with sick sinus syndrome or seizure disorders
    d. patients with gastrointestinal bleeding, a history of ulcers, or asthma
    e. all of the patients listed above should receive cholinesterase inhibitors with caution

13. Patients receiving cholinesterase inhibitors are assessed before and during therapy for improvement. Which aspects of the patient are assessed during therapy?
    a. cognitive ability
    b. functional ability
    c. physical condition
    d. only the cognitive and functional abilities are assessed
    e. cognitive, functional, and physical conditions are assessed

14. The primary use of ginseng is to _____ .
    a. decrease urinary retention
    b. increase strength
    c. improve energy and mental performance
    d. decrease inappropriate responses
    e. all of the answers are correct

15. Ginseng can have the adverse reactions of _____ .
    a. headache
    b. sleeplessness
    c. nervousness
    d. diarrhea
    e. all of the answers are correct

16. Ginseng may be contraindicated in which of the following patients?

a. type 2 diabetics, or patients taking insulin or oral antidiabetic medications
b. patients taking digoxin or warfarin sodium
c. patients who are pregnant or who have high blood pressure
d. patients taking stimulants, including caffeine
e. all of the answers are correct

17. Ginkgo biloba is most commonly used to _____ .
    a. improve symptoms associated with reduced blood flow to the brain
    b. improve short-term memory loss and dizziness
    c. treat ringing in the ears, headache, depression, and anxiety
    d. treat erectile dysfunction
    e. all of the answers are correct

18. Ginkgo biloba is contraindicated in patients who _____ .
    a. are taking monoamine oxidase inhibitors (MAOIs)
    b. are taking anticlotting medications, including aspirin
    c. are taking thiazide diuretics
    d. are taking more than one of the above medications
    e. are taking any of the above medications

19. Potential side effects of regular use of ginkgo biloba include _____ .
    a. mild GI upset
    b. headache
    c. rash
    d. muscle spasm
    e. all of the answers are correct

VI. FILL IN THE BLANK

Fill in the blanks using words from the list below.

increased	tacrine
ALT	several
mild	progressive
weight loss	eating problems

1. In the late stages of Alzheimer's disease, _____ and _____ are two major issues for patients and caregivers.

2. When ginkgo biloba is used with warfarin or vitamin E, the patient has a(n) _____ risk of bleeding.

3. Alzheimer's disease is a(n) _____ disorder.

4. Adverse reactions associated with cholinesterase inhibitors are usually _____ and generally do not last for more than _____ days.

5. Liver damage in patients taking _____ may be monitored with _____ levels.

VII. LIST

List the requested number of items

1. List four key points about taking cholinesterase inhibitors.

a. _____

b. _____

c. _____

d. _____

2. List three types of drugs used to treat Alzheimer's disease.

a. _____

b. _____

c. _____

VIII. CLINICAL APPLICATION

1. Mrs. P has been diagnosed with Alzheimer's disease. Explain to her family what potential changes to her therapy may occur if she has a poor response to one therapy.

I. MATTCHING

Match the term from Column A with the correct definition from Column B.

COLUMN A

_____ 1. antiemetic

_____ 2. nausea

_____ 3. prophylaxis

_____ 4. vertigo

_____ 5. vestibular neuritis

_____ 6. antivertigo

_____ 7. emesis

_____ 8. chemoreceptor trigger zone

COLUMN B

A. A drug used to treat or prevent nausea or vomiting.
B. An unpleasant gastric sensation usually preceding vomiting.
C. An abnormal feeling of spinning or rotation motion that may occur with motion sickness and other disorders.
D. Inflammation of the vestibular nerve to the inner ear.
E. The expelled gastric contents.
F. A drug or treatment designed for prevention of a condition or symptom.
G. A drug used to treat or prevent vertigo.
H. A group of nerve fibers in the brain that when stimulated by chemicals, sends impulses to the vomiting center of the brain.

II. MATCHING

Match the generic name of the drug in Column A with the trade name in Column B.

COLUMN A

_____ 1. chlorpromazine HCl

_____ 2. dimenhydrinate

_____ 3. diphenhydramine

_____ 4. metoclopramide

_____ 5. dronabinol

_____ 6. promethazine HCl

_____ 7. prochlorperazine HCl

_____ 8. ondansetron HCl

_____ 9. meclizine

_____ 10. transdermal scopolamine

COLUMN B

A. Dramamine, Dinate
B. Antivert
C. Phenergan
D. Compazine
E. Zofran
F. Thorazine
G. Marinol
H. Benadryl
I. Reglan
J. Transderm-Scop

III. MATCHING

Match the drug in Column A with the contraindication, precaution, or interaction in Column B.

COLUMN A

_____ 1. metoclopramide

_____ 2. prochlorperazine

_____ 3. thiethylperazine

_____ 4. promethazine

_____ 5. trimethobenzamide

_____ 6. antiemetics

_____ 7. dimenhydrinate

_____ 8. ondansetron

_____ 9. ginger

COLUMN B

A. bone marrow depression, blood dyscrasia, Parkinson's disease, severe liver disease
B. pregnancy

C. seizure disorders, breast cancer, GI obstruction, pheochromocytoma
D. hypertension, sleep apnea, epilepsy
E. ototoxic drugs
F. children with viral illnesses
G. hypertension, gallstones, morning sickness of pregnancy
H. antacids
I. rifampin

IV. TRUE/FALSE

Indicate whether each statement is True (T) or False (F).

_____ 1. An antivertigo drug is used to prevent nausea.

_____ 2. Vomiting caused by drugs, radiation, or metabolic disorders usually occurs because of stimulation of the chemoreceptor trigger zone.

_____ 3. Antiemetics are used to induce vomiting in cases of drug overdoses.

_____ 4. The most common adverse reaction of antiemetics and antivertigo drugs is varying degrees of drowsiness.

_____ 5. Thiethylperazine is contraindicated during pregnancy.

_____ 6. Ginger is classified by the FDA as a dietary supplement.

_____ 7. Patients who are being treated with antiemetics or antivertigo drugs have no alcohol restrictions.

_____ 8. Driving should be avoided while taking antiemetics or antivertigo drugs.

_____ 9. It is not a problem for patients to "share" their transdermal scopolamine patches while on a cruise because everyone is young and healthy.

V. MULTIPLE CHOICE

Circle the letter of the best answer.

1. A drug that would be more effective for vertigo associated with middle or inner ear surgery would probably act _____ .

    a. by inhibiting the chemoreceptor trigger zone in the brain
    b. by depressing the vestibular apparatus of the inner ear
    c. by sending impulses to the vomiting center in the medulla
    d. by changing the patients electrolyte balance
    e. none of the answers are correct

2. Prophylactic antiemetics are commonly given to patients _____ .

    a. before surgery
    b. before antineoplastic drug administration
    c. with bacterial or viral infections
    d. before radiation therapy
    e. all of the answers are correct

3. Antivertigo drugs are commonly used _____ .

    a. as an antiemetic
    b. to treat vertigo
    c. to treat motion sickness
    d. to prevent nausea and vomiting
    e. all of the answers are correct

4. Patients in whom antiemetics and antivertigo drugs are contraindicated include those _____ .

    a. with a known hypersensitivity to the drugs
    b. in a coma
    c. with severe CNS depression
    d. answers a and b are correct
    e. answers a, b, and c are correct

5. Antiemetic drugs may hamper the diagnosis of disorders such as _____ .

    a. brain tumors
    b. appendicitis
    c. intestinal obstruction
    d. drug toxicity
    e. all of the answers are correct

VI. RECALL FACTS

Indicate which of the following statements are Facts with an F. If the statement is not a fact, leave the line blank.

About Patient Management Issues for Antiemetics and Antivertigo Drugs

_____ 1. Dehydration is a serious concern in patients experiencing vomiting.

_____ 2. Patients may need to be weighed daily or weekly if they experience prolonged or repeated episodes of vomiting.

_____ 3. All patients experiencing vomiting should be given either a parenteral form or a rectal suppository form of antiemetic.

_____ 4. Before starting drug therapy, vital signs should be taken.

_____ 5. Elderly patients are at no higher risk for developing fluid and electrolyte disturbances caused by vomiting.

_____ 6. The odor of vomitus on soiled bedding or clothing may intensify the patient's nausea.

VII. FILL IN THE BLANK

Fill in the blanks using words from the list below.

additive	diphenidol
dehydration	diphenhydramine
antiemetics	vertigo
vital signs	dimenhydrinate
ginger	antacids

1. Elderly or chronically ill patients experiencing vomiting may develop _____ rapidly.

2. Before drug therapy begins, _____ are taken and the patient is assessed.

3. _____ may mask the signs and symptoms of ototoxicity when administered with ototoxic drugs.

4. Antiemetics and antivertigo drugs may have _____ effects when used with alcohol and other CNS depressants.

5. Antivertigo drugs are essentially the same as _____.

6. A person experiencing _____ often has trouble walking.

7. _____ decrease the absorption of the antiemetics.

8. _____ is not recommended for morning sickness associated with pregnancy.

9. The drug that is used to treat Ménière's disease is _____.

10. _____ is also used as an antihistamine.

VIII. LIST

List the requested number of items.

1. List the trade names of five antiemetic drugs that are used for patients receiving antineoplastic drug therapy.

   a. _____

   b. _____

   c. _____

   d. _____

2. List two drugs used to treat intractable hiccoughs.

   a. _____

   b. _____

3. List three drugs used to prevent and treat nausea owing to motion sickness.

   a. _____

   b. _____

   c. _____

4. List six Pregnancy Category C antiemetics and antivertigo drugs.

   a. _____

   b. _____

   c. _____

   d. _____

   e. _____

   f. _____

IX. CLINICAL APPLICATION

1. Miss Q is getting married and planning a cruise for her honeymoon trip. She knows that she experiences motion sickness when she travels and has come to her healthcare provider to get a prescription to prevent this event from marring her honeymoon. What should Miss Q be aware of regarding the use of antivertigo drugs in general?

9 Anesthetic Drugs

I. MATCHING

Match the term from Column A with the correct definition from Column B.

COLUMN A

_____ 1. analgesia

_____ 2. anesthesia

_____ 3. atelectasis

_____ 4. conduction block

_____ 5. general anesthesia

_____ 6. local anesthesia

_____ 7. patency

_____ 8. regional anesthesia

COLUMN B

A. Being open or exposed.
B. Provision of a pain-free state for the entire body.
C. Reduction of air in the lungs.
D. Absence of pain.
E. Anesthesia produced by injecting a local anesthetic around nerves to limit the pain signals sent to the brain.
F. Provision of a pain-free state in a specific area.
G. Type of regional anesthesia produced by injection of a local anesthetic into or near a nerve trunk.
H. A loss of feeling or sensation.

II. MATCHING

Match the type of anesthesia in Column A with the injection site in Column B.

COLUMN A

_____ 1. topical

_____ 2. local infiltration

_____ 3. regional

_____ 4. spinal

_____ 5. epidural block

_____ 6. transsacral block

_____ 7. brachial plexus

COLUMN B

A. Subarachnoid space of the spinal cord (L2).
B. Brachial plexus.
C. Epidural space at the level of sacrococcygeal notch.
D. In tissues.
E. The surface of the skin, open area, or mucous membrane.
F. The space surrounding the dura of the spinal cord.
G. Around nerves.

III. MATCHING

Match the stage number of general surgical anesthesia in Column A with the description in Column B.

COLUMN A

_____ 1. Stage 1

_____ 2. Stage 2

_____ 3. Stage 3

_____ 4. Stage 4

COLUMN B

A. Surgical anesthesia.
B. Induction—lasts until patient loses consciousness.
C. Respiratory paralysis.
D. Delirium and excitement.

IV. MATCHING

Match the anesthetic drug listed in Column A with the correct anesthetic classification from Column B. You may use an answer more than once.

COLUMN A

_____ 1. lidocaine HCl

_____ 2. tubocurarine chloride

_____ 3. atracurium besylate

_____ 4. scopolamine

_____ 5. tetracaine HCl

_____ 6. fentanyl

_____ 7. diazepam

_____ 8. procaine HCl

_____ 9. metocurine iodine

COLUMN B

A. Pre-anesthetic
B. Local anesthetic
C. Muscle relaxant used during general anesthesia

V. MATCHING

Match the type of anesthesia commonly used in Column A with the procedure listed in Column B. You may use an answer more than once.

COLUMN A

_____ 1. topical

_____ 2. local infiltration

_____ 3. epidural block

_____ 4. transsacral block

_____ 5. brachial plexus block

COLUMN B

A. Hand surgery
B. Obstetrics
C. Desensitize skin for injection of local anesthesia
D. Tissue sample for biopsy

VI. TRUE/FALSE

Indicate whether each statement is True (T) or False (F).

_____ 1. The two types of anesthesia are regional and spinal.

_____ 2. Spinal anesthesia and conduction blocks are two types of regional anesthesia.

_____ 3. A pre-anesthetic drug is only used before the administration of a general anesthetic.

_____ 4. A pre-anesthetic drug may be given up to 2 hours before surgery.

_____ 5. Cholinergic blocking drugs are used as pre-anesthetic drugs because they de-

crease the secretions of the upper respiratory tract.

_____ 6. During the administration of general anesthesia, reflexes such as the swallowing and gag reflex are lost.

_____ 7. IV and IM methods of administration are most commonly used for general anesthetics.

_____ 8. Anesthesia begins with the loss of consciousness.

_____ 9. Nitrous oxide is the most commonly used anesthetic gas.

_____ 10. Methohexital and thiopental do not produce analgesia.

VII. MULTIPLE CHOICE

Circle the letter of the best answer.

1. A patient receiving local anesthesia _____ .
   a. never requires sedation
   b. often has no memory of the procedure
   c. has had many pre-anesthetic drugs
   d. is fully awake but does not feel pain in the area that has been anesthetized
   e. none of the answers are correct

2. Examples of conduction block anesthetics include all of the following except _____ .
   a. epidural
   b. spinal
   c. transsacral
   d. brachial plexus
   e. all of the answers are correct

3. Preparing a patient for local anesthesia may involve _____ .
   a. an allergy history
   b. prepping the body area for the procedure
   c. giving the patient a sedative
   d. an explanation of the administration of the anesthetic
   e. all of the answers are correct

4. Which of the following can be used as pre-anesthetic drugs?
   a. narcotics
   b. cholinergic blocking drugs
   c. antianxiety drugs
   d. antiemetics
   e. all of the answers are correct

5. A general anesthetic produces _____ .
   a. a pain-free state for the entire body
   b. a pain-free state for a part of the body
   c. a loss of consciousness
   d. answers a and c are correct
   e. answers a, b, and c are correct

6. Which of the following drugs is a nonbarbiturate used for induction of anesthesia?
   a. etomidate
   b. ketamine
   c. midazolam
   d. ethylene
   e. isoflurane

7. During general anesthesia a skeletal muscle relaxant, such as _____, may be used to facilitate intubation of the patient or relax skeletal muscles for surgical procedures.
   a. chlordiazepoxide
   b. rapacuronium bromide
   c. morphine sulfate
   d. ropivacaine
   e. sevoflurane

8. Antiemetics are used to prevent _____ during the immediate postoperative recovery period.
   a. nausea and vomiting
   b. diarrhea and gastric upset
   c. vertigo
   d. drooling and coughing
   e. dry mouth and wheezing

9. Droperidol may be used _____ .
   a. alone as a tranquilizer
   b. as an antiemetic in the immediate postanesthesia period
   c. as an induction drug
   d. as an adjunct to general anesthesia
   e. all of the answers are correct

10. _____ is used for continuous sedation of intubated or respiratory-controlled patients in intensive care units.
    a. Etomidate
    b. Ketamine
    c. Propofol
    d. Midazolam
    e. Ethylene

VIII. RECALL FACTS

Indicate which of the following statements are Facts with an F. If the statement is not a fact, leave the line blank.

About Drugs Used for Induction and Maintenance of Anesthesia

_____ 1. cyclopropane

_____ 2. enflurane

_____ 3. nitrous oxide

_____ 4. sevoflurane

_____ 5. halothane

_____ 6. propofol

_____ 7. ethylene

_____ 8. ketamine

_____ 9. isoflurane

_____ 10. midazolam

_____ 11. desflurane

_____ 12. remifentanil HCl

IX. FILL IN THE BLANK

Fill in the blanks using words from the list below.

neuroleptanalgesia   inhaled analgesic
etomidate   methohexital
thiopental   Innovar
explosive   decrease

1. Sublimaze and Inapsine when used together as a single drug are called _____ .

2. Cyclopropane and ethylene when used mixed with oxygen are _____ .

3. Innovar results in _____ .

4. Sevoflurane is an _____ .

5. _____ is a nonbarbiturate used for induction of anesthesia.

6 and 7. _____ and

_____ are ultra-short-acting barbi-

turates that depress the CNS to produce hypnosis

and anesthesia.

8. Cholinergic blocking drugs are used

to _____ secretions of the upper

respiratory tract.

X. LIST

List the requested number of items.

1. List five examples of a volatile liquid anesthetic.

    a. _____

    b. _____

    c. _____

    d. _____

    e. _____

2. List five uses of local anesthetics.

    a. _____

    b. _____

    c. _____

    d. _____

    e. _____

3. List four reasons to use a pre-anesthetic drug.

    a. _____

    b. _____

    c. _____

    d. _____

4. List three factors that help determine the choice of anesthetic drug used for general anesthesia.

    a. _____

    b. _____

    c. _____

XI. CLINICAL APPLICATION

1. The healthcare provider for whom you work has recommended surgery using general anesthesia for Mrs. Y's hysterectomy. Please explain to the patient the different stages of anesthesia she will undergo during this procedure.

I. MATTCHING

Match the term from Column A with the correct definition from Column B.

COLUMN A

_____ 1. agonist

_____ 2. antagonist

_____ 3. antipyretic

_____ 4. miosis

_____ 5. opioids

_____ 6. partial agonist

_____ 7. salicylates

_____ 8. tinnitus

COLUMN B

A. A category of narcotic analgesic that binds to a receptor but has a limited response.
B. Pinpoint pupils.
C. Narcotic analgesics obtained from the opium plant.
D. A category of narcotic analgesic that binds to a receptor and causes a response.
E. Drugs that have analgesic antipyretic and anti-inflammatory effects.
F. Ringing sound in the ear.
G. A drug that reduces elevated body temperature.
H. A substance that counteracts the action of something else.

II. MATCHING

Match the salicylate level in Column A with the symptoms in Column B.

COLUMN A

_____ 1. greater than 150 μg/mL

_____ 2. greater than 250 μg/mL

_____ 3. greater than 400 μg/mL

COLUMN B

A. Respiratory alkalosis, hemorrhage, fever, coma, shock
B. Tinnitus, dizziness, nausea, vomiting, hyperventilation
C. Headache, diarrhea, thirst, flushing

III. MATCHING

Match the generic salicylate or nonsalicylate in Column A to the trade name in Column B.

_____ 1. salsalate

_____ 2. acetylsalicylic acid

_____ 3. sodium thiosalicylate

_____ 4. diflunisal

_____ 5. acetaminophen

_____ 6. magnesium salicylate

_____ 7. choline salicylate

_____ 8. buffered aspirin

COLUMN B

A. Ascriptin
B. Extra Strength Doan's
C. Dolobid
D. Bayer
E. Rexolate
F. Amigesic
G. Arthropan
H. Tylenol

IV. MATCHING

Match the generic NSAID in Column A with the trade name in Column B.

COLUMN A

_____ 1. celecoxib

_____ 2. ibuprofen

_____ 3. indomethacin

_____ 4. flurbiprofen

_____ 5. sulindac

_____ 6. naproxen

_____ 7. oxaprozin

_____ 8. meloxicam

_____ 9. ketorolac

_____ 10. nabumetone

COLUMN B

A. Ansaid
B. Clinoril
C. Daypro
D. Celebrex
E. Mobic
F. Aleve, Anaprox
G. Indocin
H. Advil, Motrin
 I. Relafen
 J. Toradol

V. MATCHING

Match the generic narcotic analgesic in Column A with the trade name in Column B.

_____ 1. meperidine

_____ 2. buprenorphine

_____ 3. hydromorphone

_____ 4. morphine sulfate

_____ 5. oxymorphone

_____ 6. oxycodone

_____ 7. propoxyphene

_____ 8. fentanyl

_____ 9. methadone

_____ 10. butorphanol

COLUMN B

A. MS Contin
B. Dolophine
C. Sulimaze
D. OxyContin
E. Dilaudid
F. Stadol
G. Demerol
H. Numorphan
 I. Darvon
 J. Buprenex

VI. MATCHING

Match the trade name in Column A to the category of drug in Column B. You may use an answer more than once.

COLUMN A

_____ 1. Stadol

_____ 2. Alfenta

_____ 3. Talwin

_____ 4. Buprenex

_____ 5. Levo-Dromoran

_____ 6. Orlaam

_____ 7. Nubain

_____ 8. Ultiva

COLUMN B

A. Agonist
B. Partial agonist
C. Agonist antagonist

VII. TRUE/FALSE

Indicate whether each statement is True (T) or False (F).

_____ 1. Nonnarcotic analgesics are used to relieve pain and have the possibility of causing physical dependency.

_____ 2. The analgesic action of salicylates is owed to inhibition of prostaglandin.

_____ 3. Salicylism is caused by salicylate toxicity and is reversible with a reduction in dosage.

_____ 4. Tinnitus or impaired hearing caused by high blood salicylate levels will not disappear once the drug is discontinued.

_____ 5. Acetaminophen is the only nonsalicylate available in the United States.

_____ 6. Acetaminophen is widely used for its anti-inflammatory action.

_____ 7. Chronic alcoholics may safely take acetaminophen but should avoid NSAIDs.

_____ 8. The goal of acetaminophen therapy is relief of pain.

_____ 9. The NSAIDs have anti-inflammatory, antipyretic, and analgesic effects.

_____ 10. Patients may take salicylates or acetaminophen with food.

_____ 11. NSAIDs are nonnarcotic analgesics.

_____ 12. NSAIDs act by inhibiting the action of the enzyme cyclooxygenase.

_____ 13. When monitoring a patient taking an NSAID, the healthcare provider need only be notified if active bleeding occurs.

_____ 14. Age appears to increase the incidence of adverse reactions to NSAIDs.

_____ 15. Narcotic analgesics are classified as non-agonists, antagonists, or mixed agonists.

_____ 16. Morphine is a model narcotic.

_____ 17. A major hazard of narcotic analgesic administration is respiratory depression.

_____ 18. Older adults may require a lower dosage of a narcotic analgesic.

_____ 19. Newborns of an opiate-dependent mother may exhibit signs of withdrawal during the first few days after birth.

_____ 20. In patient-controlled analgesia, it is easy for patients to accidentally overdose themselves.

_____ 21. OxyContin is an effective and safe drug for use in elderly patients because patients tend to have fewer adverse reactions than with morphine.

_____ 22. Naloxone can be used to reverse the effects of a narcotic if needed.

_____ 23. Patients using narcotics for severe pain often become addicted to the drug.

_____ 24. Naloxone is a narcotic antagonist that can abruptly reverse a narcotic depression.

_____ 25. Naltrexone use may inhibit the action of opioid antidiarrheals, antitussives, and analgesics.

VIII. MULTIPLE CHOICE

Circle the letter of the best answer.

1. All of the following are types of nonnarcotic analgesic drugs except _____ .
   a. salicylates
   b. partial agonists
   c. nonsalicylates
   d. nonsteroidal anti-inflammatory drugs
   e. all of the answers are correct

2. Salicylates act to have an _____ effect.
   a. analgesic
   b. antipyretic
   c. anesthetic
   d. anti-inflammatory
   e. answers a, b, and d are correct

3. Long-term salicylate use by older adults can lead to _____ .
   a. addiction
   b. a reduction in the effectiveness of the drug
   c. gastrointestinal bleeding
   d. permanent hearing loss
   e. Reye's syndrome

4. Salicylates are contraindicated in all of the following patients except _____ .
   a. patients receiving NSAID therapy
   b. pregnant women
   c. patients with bleeding disorders
   d. children or teenagers with influenza or chickenpox
   e. patients receiving antineoplastic drugs

5. _____ is the salicylate that can be given by the IM route.
   a. Choline salicylate
   b. Sodium thiosalicylate
   c. Diflunisal
   d. Salsalate
   e. Magnesium salicylate

6. Acetaminophen _____ .
   a. is the drug of choice for treating children with fever and flu-like symptoms
   b. has analgesic activities
   c. has antipyretic activities
   d. has anti-inflammatory activities
   e. answers a, b, and c are correct

7. Excessive doses of acetaminophen can cause _____ .
   a. necrosis of liver cells
   b. hemophilia
   c. gastrointestinal bleeding
   d. respiratory distress
   e. all of the answers are correct

8. Miss C has been taking acetaminophen for her osteoarthritis. Lately the drug has not been as effective, so Miss C has increased her dose to 12 g/day. As the healthcare worker taking care of her, what might you be watching for at this dose level?

a. nausea and vomiting
b. anorexia
c. abdominal pain
d. jaundice
e. all of the answers are correct

9. What should a patient avoid while taking acetaminophen?

a. alcohol consumption
b. salicylates
c. NSAIDs
d. answers a and c are correct
e. all of the answers are correct

10. Miss G complains about the fact that before and after her dental surgery she is not to take her usual dose of salicylates for her arthritis. What might her healthcare provider suggest she take to relieve her pain and decrease the inflammation?

a. ibuprofen
b. acetaminophen
c. naproxen
d. mefenamic acid
e. answers a, c, and d are correct

11. Celecoxib relieves pain without causing gastrointestinal upset because it selectively inhibits _____ .

a. prostaglandin synthesis
b. cyclooxygenase-2 (COX-2)
c. cyclooxygenase-1 (COX-1)
d. both COX-1 and COX -2
e. none of the answers are correct

12. Adverse reactions of NSAIDs can include _____ .

a. nausea and vomiting
b. dizziness and vertigo
c. cardiac arrhythmias
d. skin rashes and ecchymoses
e. all of the answers are correct

13. Of the following drugs, which is (are) available over-the-counter?

a. sulindac
b. celecoxib
c. naproxen
d. ibuprofen
e. answers c and d are correct

14. Patients who should not take any type of NSAID include those who are _____ .

a. allergic to porcine products
b. sensitive to narcotics
c. hypersensitive to aspirin

d. experiencing flu-like symptoms
e. have had a myocardial infarction

15. Narcotic analgesics _____ .

a. are used to manage moderate to severe acute and chronic pain
b. lessen anxiety and sedation
c. provide obstetrical analgesia
d. relieve pain from a heart attack
e. all of the answers are correct

16. In which of the following situations should the narcotic analgesic be withheld from a patient and the healthcare provider contacted immediately?

a. An increase in the respiratory rate
b. A significant decrease in the respiratory rate or a rate of 10 breaths/min or less
c. A significant increase or decrease in the pulse rate
d. A significant decrease in the blood pressure or a systolic pressure less than 100 mm Hg.
e. Answers b, c, and d are correct.

17. Signs that a patient is developing a dependence on a narcotic include all of the following except _____ .

a. withdrawal symptoms
b. frequent requests for the narcotic
c. personality changes when drug is not received
d. anorexia and weight loss
e. complaints of pain or failure of drug to relieve pain

18. A patient who has been using or abusing narcotics may experience _____ when given an agonist-antagonist narcotic analgesic.

a. a synergistic effect
b. withdrawal symptoms
c. no difference in effectiveness
d. a decreased effectiveness
e. none of the answers are correct

19. An increased risk of respiratory depression can occur with narcotic analgesic use _____ .

a. when they are administered too soon after barbiturate anesthesia
b. in older adults
c. in obese patients
d. in neonates
e. all of the answers are correct

20. By which routes can morphine be administered?

a. orally and rectally
b. subcutaneously

c. intramuscularly
d. intravenously
e. all of the answers are correct

21. Epidural administration of narcotic analgesics has all of the following advantages except _____ .

   a. fewer adverse reactions
   b. lower total dosage of drug
   c. greater patient comfort
   d. more adverse reactions
   e. direct effect on opiate receptors

22. Passion flower when used as an herbal remedy has all of the following qualities except _____ .

   a. has no reported adverse reactions
   b. is thought to have calming qualities
   c. is contraindicated in pregnancy
   d. is available in the U.S. as an over-the-counter sedative
   e. can increase the risk of bleeding in patients taking warfarin

23. Naloxone _____ .

   a. is used to prevent the effects of opiates in the treatment of narcotic-dependent patients
   b. can restore respiratory function in 1 to 2 minutes
   c. has no activity if no opiates have been taken
   d. can be used to diagnose a suspected opioid overdosage
   e. all of the answers are correct

24. All of the following statements about naltrexone are correct except one. Which is the exception?

   a. Naltrexone completely blocks the effects of IV opiates.
   b. Naltrexone is used to treat patients dependent on opioids.
   c. Naltrexone alone will keep patients in an opioid-free state.
   d. Patients being treated with naltrexone have been detoxified and are enrolled in a treatment program.
   e. If taking naltrexone on a scheduled basis, opiate us will have no narcotic effect.

IX. RECALL FACTS

Indicate which of the following statements are Facts with an F. If the statement is not a fact, leave the line blank.

About Uses for Salicylates

_____ 1. Relief of mild to moderate pain

_____ 2. Decreased risk of MI in certain patients

_____ 3. Decreased risk of TIA or strokes caused by fibrin platelet emboli in men

_____ 4. Relief of pain associated with cancer

_____ 5. Relief of bacterial endotoxin tissue damage

_____ 6. Reduction of elevated body temperature

_____ 7. Treatment of inflammatory conditions

About Adverse Reactions Caused by Long-Term Use of Acetaminophen

_____ 1. Hemolytic anemia

_____ 2. Respiratory depression

_____ 3. Hypoglycemia

_____ 4. Skin eruptions or urticaria

_____ 5. Hepatotoxicity

_____ 6. Elevated blood pressure

About Acetaminophen Toxicity Treatment

_____ 1. Gastric lavage

_____ 2. Antacids prescribed

_____ 3. Liver function tests

_____ 4. Acetylcysteine prescribed

_____ 5. Airway management

_____ 6. Syrup of ipecac prescribed

About Synthetic Analgesics

_____ 1. hydromorphone

_____ 2. methadone

_____ 3. oxymorphone

_____ 4. levorphanol

_____ 5. remifentanil

_____ 6. oxycodone

_____ 7. meperidine

About Patients in Whom All Narcotic Analgesics Are Contraindicated

_____ 1. osteoarthritis

_____ 2. known hypersensitivity

_____ 3. acute bronchial asthma

_____ 4. myocardial infarction

_____ 5. upper airway obstruction

_____ 6. head injury

_____ 7. increased intracranial pressure

_____ 8. recent dental surgery

_____ 9. convulsive disorders

_____ 10. renal or hepatic dysfunction

_____ 11. Reye's syndrome

_____ 12. acute ulcerative colitis

X. FILL IN THE BLANK

Fill in the blanks using words from the list below. You may use a word more than once.

depressed	PRN
lower	decrease
one	COX-2
COX-1	increase
fewer	greater
high	ibuprofen
methadone	scheduled
agonist	antagonist
levomethadyl	naproxen
celecoxib	

1. Aspirin has a(n) _____ anti-inflammatory effect and a(n) _____ effect on platelets than do other salicylates, and also has a(n) _____ inhibitory effect on prostaglandin synthesis.

2. Willow bark has _____ adverse reactions than salicylates and must be taken in _____ doses to have an effect.

3. Acetaminophen may _____ blood glucose values.

4. Patients should discontinue salicylate therapy at least _____ week(s) before any type of surgery.

5. To prevent gastric upset, patients may take salicylates or acetaminophen _____ food or water.

6. The anti-inflammatory effects of NSAIDs are due to the inhibition of _____, whereas the gastrointestinal adverse reactions are due to blocking of _____ .

7. NSAIDs can prolong bleeding time and _____ the effects of anticoagulants, but can _____ the effects of antihypertensive drugs.

8. _____ is contraindicated in patients allergic to sulfonamides.

9. _____ and _____ increase the risk of lithium toxicity in patients taking both drugs.

10. The two opioids used for the treatment and management of opiate dependency are _____ and _____ .

11. Narcotic analgesic adverse reactions differ according to whether the narcotic acts as a(n) _____ or a(n) _____ .

12. When adverse reactions to narcotic analgesics occur, the healthcare provider may _____ the dose in an effort to _____ the intensity of the reaction.

13. The cough reflex of a patient taking a narcotic may be _____ .

14. Morphine, when used to treat chronic pain, such as in cancer, is not given on

    a _____ basis but on

    a _____ basis.

XI. LIST

List the requested number of items.

1. List the three types of pain.

    a. _____

    b. _____

    c. _____

2. List four examples of salicylates by trade name.

    a. _____

    b. _____

    c. _____

    d. _____

3. List six adverse reactions associated with salicylates.

    a. _____

    b. _____

    c. _____

    d. _____

    e. _____

    f. _____

4. List four conditions in which patients may find acetaminophen treatment useful.

    a. _____

    b. _____

    c. _____

    d. _____

5. List four uses of NSAIDs.

    a. _____

    b. _____

    c. _____

    d. _____

6. List the three receptors that are involved in the actions of narcotic analgesics.

    a. _____

    b. _____

    c. _____

7. List six factors that determine the ability of a narcotic analgesic to relieve pain.

    a. _____

    b. _____

    c. _____

    d. _____

    e. _____

    f. _____

8. List five drugs that may be included in Brompton's mixture.

    a. _____

    b. _____

    c. _____

    d. _____

    e. _____

XII. CLINICAL APPLICATIONS

1. Mr. G will be taking an NSAID as part of his treatment program. What information should the healthcare provider make sure that Mr. G knows about these drugs?

2. Mrs. Z has had a surgical procedure and has been placed on a PCA infusion pump. What should Mrs. Z have been instructed about the pump before its use?

11 Antihistamines and Decongestants

I. MATCHING

Match the term from Column A with the correct definition from Column B.

COLUMN A

_____ 1. antihistamine

_____ 2. epigastric disorder

_____ 3. expectoration

_____ 4. histamine

_____ 5. rebound

COLUMN B

A. The elimination of thick, tenacious mucus from the respiratory tract by spitting it up.
B. Discomfort in the abdomen.
C. A substance in various body tissues, such as the heart, lungs, gastric mucosa, and skin, that is produced in response to injury.
D. A drug used to counteract the effects of histamine on body organs and structures.
E. Causing the opposite of the desired effect.

II. MATCHING

Match the generic antihistamine or decongestant in Column A with the trade name in Column B.

COLUMN A

_____ 1. loratadine

_____ 2. diphenhydramine

_____ 3. fexofenadine

_____ 4. cetirizine

_____ 5. desloratadine

_____ 6. fluticasone propionate

_____ 7. triamcinolone acetonide

_____ 8. phenylephrine

_____ 9. oxymetazoline

_____ 10. pseudoephedrine

_____ 11. hydroxyzine

_____ 12. naphazoline HCl

_____ 13. tetrahydrozoline HCl

_____ 14. ephedrine

_____ 15. clemastine fumarate

COLUMN B

A. Zyrtec
B. Benadryl
C. Neo-Synephrine
D. Atarax
E. Allegra
F. Nasacort AQ
G. Afrin
H. Claritin
I. Flonase
J. Pertz-D
K. Tavist
L. Clarinex
M. Privine
N. Tyzine
O. Sudafed

III. TRUE/FALSE

Indicate whether each statement is True (T) or False (F).

_____ 1. Histamine release produces localized redness and swelling at the site of an injury.

_____ 2. Some antihistamines are able to prevent vomiting.

_____ 3. Antihistamines may be taken by a woman who is nursing an infant with no adverse effect to the infant.

_____ 4. Most antihistamines are administered topically.

_____ 5. Respiratory secretions may become thickened because of the use of antihistamines.

_____ 6. An adverse reaction of oral decongestants may be tachycardia and insomnia.

IV. MULTIPLE CHOICE

Circle the letter of the best answer.

1. Histamine _____ .

    a. release produces an inflammatory response
    b. is released in allergic reactions
    c. is released in anaphylactic shock
    d. produces increased vasodilation and increased capillary permeability
    e. all of the answers are correct

2. Miss T is experiencing an allergic reaction to a bee sting. As a result, she might _____ .

    a. need to take a histamine stimulant
    b. need to use an antihistamine
    c. go into anaphylactic shock
    d. answers b and c are correct
    e. all of the answers are correct

3. Antihistamines have an action of _____ .

    a. stimulating histamine receptors
    b. increasing the release of histamine by mast cells and basophils
    c. competing with histamine for receptor sites
    d. completely blocking all histamine receptor sites
    e. blocking the release of histamine by mast cells and basophils

4. After taking an antihistamine for several days for his seasonal allergy, Mr. J is starting to itch and has a rash on his chest. He may _____ .

    a. be experiencing an adverse reaction
    b. be becoming used to the drug
    c. need to increase the dose he is taking
    d. be developing an allergy to the antihistamine
    e. none of the answers are correct

5. Which of the following is an oral nasal decongestant?

    a. loratadine
    b. diphenhydramine
    c. fluticasone propionate
    d. pseudoephedrine
    e. phenylephedrine

6. Which of the following effects might Miss T experience as a result of the anticholinergic effects of her antihistamine medication?

    a. dry mouth, nose, and throat
    b. dizziness, fatigue, and hypotension
    c. photosensitivity
    d. skin rash and urticaria
    e. anaphylactic shock

7. Nasal decongestants _____ .

    a. are sympathomimetic drugs
    b. produce localized vasoconstriction
    c. come in topical or oral forms
    d. answers b and c are correct
    e. answers a, b, and c are correct

8. Miss A, who is 82 years old, has been prescribed an antihistamine. Which of the following might Miss A be likely to experience as a result of this medication?

    a. nervousness and irritability
    b. dizziness, sedation, and hypotension
    c. speech difficulties
    d. anticholinergic effects
    e. answers b and d are correct

9. Of the following patients, which one is not a candidate for a decongestant?

    a. a patient taking a MAOI
    b. a hypotensive patient
    c. a patient with severe coronary artery disease
    d. answers a and c are correct.
    e. decongestant use is contraindicated in all of these patients

10. Mrs. S is experiencing rebound nasal congestion as a result of overuse. What might you suggest to her to minimize the adverse reaction?

    a. Stop using the nasal decongestants immediately.
    b. Continue using the nasal decongestants as often as needed, as this reaction will go away in time.
    c. Gradually discontinue use in one nostril and then the other.
    d. Decrease use in both nostrils by 1 time per day.
    e. She is now addicted and will always need to use the nasal decongestant.

V. FILL IN THE BLANK

Fill in the blanks using words from the list below.

hypertension	heart disease
naphazoline	antihistamines
drowsiness	sedation
antiemetic	antipruritic
contraindicated	topical
oral	nasal decongestant
MAOI	stinging sensation

1. Antihistamines may have additional effects such as _____, _____, or sedative effects.

2. Common adverse reactions of many antihistamines are _____ and _____.

3. Antihistamines are _____ in lactating women since the drugs pass readily into breast milk.

4. _____ should not be taken by patients with lower respiratory tract diseases, including asthma.

5. _____ application of decongestants is more effective than the _____ route.

6. _____ is contraindicated in patients with glaucoma.

7. Use of a(n) _____ along with a(n) _____ may cause a hypertensive crisis.

8. Nonprescription nasal decongestants should not be used by patients with _____ or _____ unless approved by their healthcare provider.

9. After using a topical nasal decongestant, some patients may experience a mild _____, which usually disappears with continued use.

VI. LIST

List the requested number of items.

1. List eight uses of antihistamines.

   a. _____

   b. _____

   c. _____

   d. _____

   e. _____

   f. _____

   g. _____

   h. _____

2. List five types of patients in whom antihistamines are used with caution.

   a. _____

   b. _____

   c. _____

   d. _____

   e. _____

3. List six uses of decongestants.

   a. _____

   b. _____

   c. _____

   d. _____

   e. _____

   f. _____

VII. CLINICAL APPLICATIONS

1. Explain to Miss E why overusing her nasal decongestant can lead to rebound nasal congestion.

2. To help Mr. W get the maximum benefit from using a decongestant, what should you, as his healthcare worker, be sure that he knows about this medication?

12 Bronchodilators and Antiasthma Drugs

I. MATCHING

Match the term from Column A with the correct definition from Column B.

COLUMN A

_____ 1. sympathomimetics

_____ 2. theophyllinization

_____ 3. leukotrienes

_____ 4. xanthine derivatives

_____ 5. emphysema

_____ 6. chronic bronchitis

_____ 7. dyspnea

_____ 8. bronchiectasis

COLUMN B

A. Substances that are released by the body during the inflammatory process and constrict the bronchia.
B. A lung disorder in which the terminal bronchioles or alveoli become enlarged and plugged with mucus.
C. Difficulty breathing.
D. Drugs that mimic the activities of the sympathetic nervous system.
E. Abnormal condition of the bronchial tree.
F. Abnormal inflammation and possible infection of the bronchi.
G. Process of giving the patient a higher initial dose of a prescription drug to bring drug levels of theophylline to a therapeutic range more quickly.
H. Drugs that stimulate the central nervous system and result in bronchodilation.

II. MATCHING

Match the generic corticosteroid, leukotriene, or mast cell stabilizer in Column A with the correct trade name in Column B.

COLUMN A

_____ 1. budesonide

_____ 2. flunisolide

_____ 3. beclomethasone dipropionate

_____ 4. triamcinolone

_____ 5. cromolyn

_____ 6. fluticasone propionate

_____ 7. zileuton

_____ 8. zafirlukast

_____ 9. montelukast sodium

_____ 10. nedocromil

COLUMN B

A. Pulmicort
B. Flovent
C. Singulair
D. Zyflo
E. AeroBid
F. Beconase AQ
G. Azmacort
H. Accolate
 I. Nasalcrom
J. Tilade

III. MATCHING

Match the drug in Column A with the correct classification in Column B. You may use an answer more than once.

COLUMN A

_____ 1. albuterol sulfate

_____ 2. epinephrine

_____ 3. theophylline

_____ 4. dyphylline

_____ 5. metaproterenol sulfate

_____ 6. salmeterol

_____ 7. aminophylline

_____ 8. terbutaline

_____ 9. bitolterol mesylate

_____ 10. oxtriphylline

_____ 11. salmeterol

_____ 12. isoetharine

COLUMN B

A. xanthine derivative
B. sympathomimetic

IV. TRUE/FALSE

Indicate whether each statement is True (T) or False (F).

_____ 1. Asthma is an irreversible obstructive disease of the lower airway.

_____ 2. Excessive use of an inhaled sympathomimetic bronchodilator can result in paradoxical bronchospasm.

_____ 3. Additive adrenergic effects can occur when two sympathomimetic drugs are used concurrently.

_____ 4. Xanthine derivatives stimulate the central nervous system, resulting in bronchodilation caused by relaxation of the smooth muscles in the bronchi.

_____ 5. Inhalation is the route of administration used most often for corticosteroids.

_____ 6. Vertigo, headaches, and oral fungal infections are adverse reactions of corticosteroids.

_____ 7. Montelukast works by stimulating leukotriene receptor sites in the respiratory tract.

_____ 8. Leukotriene receptor antagonists and leukotriene formation inhibitors are the drugs of choice during an acute asthma attack.

_____ 9. Zileuton therapy management includes regular monitoring of the patient's ALT levels.

_____ 10. Zileuton is contraindicated in patients with active liver disease.

_____ 11. Mast cell stabilizers act by inhibiting mast cells from releasing substances that stimulate inflammation and bronchoconstriction.

_____ 12. Mast cell stabilizers are contraindicated in patients during an acute asthma attack.

V. MULTIPLE CHOICE

Circle the letter of the best answer.

1. Allergic asthma _____.
    a. causes the release of histamine
    b. causes carbon dioxide to be trapped in the alveoli
    c. causes the production of immunoglobulin E
    d. can be triggered by an allergen
    e. all of the answers are correct

2. Bronchodilators are drugs that are used to relieve bronchospasm caused by _____.
    a. emphysema
    b. bronchial pneumonia
    c. chronic bronchitis
    d. bronchial asthma
    e. answers a, b, and d are correct

3. The nervousness, anxiety, and restlessness observed in patients who are being treated for difficulty breathing with a sympathomimetic may be caused by _____.
    a. environmental factors
    b. the respiratory disorder itself
    c. an adverse drug reaction
    d. answers b and c are correct
    e. answers a, b, and c are correct

4. Salmeterol is contraindicated in _____.
    a. patients with depression
    b. acute bronchospasm
    c. congestive heart failure
    d. renal failure
    e. none of the answers are correct

5. Theophyllinization _____.
    a. is used for acute respiratory situations
    b. uses xanthine derivatives
    c. involves giving the patient a loading dose of theophylline
    d. answers a and c are correct
    e. answers a, b, and c are correct

6. Mrs. A has been taking theophylline for her respiratory disorder. As the healthcare worker assigned to her, what might you tell Mrs. A to help her minimize possible adverse reactions from this medication?
    a. lay in a prone position
    b. remain upright and sleep with the head of the bed elevated

c. walking increases the effectiveness of the drug

d. skipping doses minimizes adverse reactions because the body has time to recover between doses

e. none of the answers are correct

7. Patients taking theophylline _____.

   a. should not drink coffee before having a theophylline blood level drawn
   b. should be monitored for toxicity
   c. may miss doses since the drug levels are stable once established
   d. can be pregnant with no risk to the fetus
   e. answers a and b are correct

8. In which of the following patients would administration of a xanthine derivative be contraindicated?

   a. a patient with a peptic ulcer
   b. a pregnant patient
   c. an elderly patient (older than 60 years of age)
   d. a patient who has hypothyroidism
   e. a patient with congestive heart failure

9. Corticosteroids that are used to manage chronic asthma or allergic rhinitis generally act by _____.

   a. increasing the sensitivity of beta-2 receptors
   b. decreasing the inflammatory response
   c. making the beta-2 receptor agonist drugs more effective
   d. answers a and c are correct
   e. answers a, b, and c are correct

10. Which of the following drugs inhibit the production of leukotrienes?

    a. montelukast
    b. zileuton
    c. cromolyn
    d. zafirlukast
    e. flunisolide

11. The common adverse reaction of headache and abdominal pain can be associated with which of the following drugs?

    a. zafirlukast
    b. montelukast
    c. zileuton
    d. answers a and c are correct
    e. answers a, b, and c are correct

12. Mr. P has been prescribed zafirlukast. Which medications should he avoid so that his plasma level of zafirlukast is not increased because of a drug interaction?

    a. warfarin sodium
    b. theophylline
    c. aspirin
    d. propanolol
    e. erythromycin

13. Mast cell stabilizers _____.

    a. may be given as an aerosol, oral concentrate, or by nebulization
    b. must be discontinued gradually
    c. can enable other antiasthma drugs to be taken in a reduced dose
    d. can be used to treat exercise-induced bronchospasm
    e. all of the answers are correct

VI. RECALL FACTS

Indicate which of the following statements are Facts with an F. If the statement is not a fact, leave the line blank.

About Things That Decrease the Effectiveness of Xanthine Derivatives

_____ 1. Citrus fruit consumption

_____ 2. Charcoal-broiled foods

_____ 3. Cigarettes

_____ 4. Coffee, colas, or chocolate

_____ 5. Isoniazid or rifampin administration

_____ 6. Pregnancy and lactation

_____ 7. Barbiturate administration

About Treatment with Sympathomimetics

_____ 1. Patients should not exceed recommended doses.

_____ 2. Tend to cause drowsiness and sedation.

_____ 3. May cause nervousness, insomnia, and restlessness.

_____ 4. Tachycardia, palpitations, and muscle tremors are normal and will pass with time.

_____ 5. Difficulty with urination or breathing should be reported to the healthcare provider.

_____ 6. Salmeterol is used for acute asthma symptoms.

_____ 7. The route of administration for formoterol fumarate is oral inhalation.

_____ 8. The regular use of short-acting beta-2 agonists is to be continued during formoterol fumarate treatment.

VII. FILL IN THE BLANK

Fill in the blanks using words from the list below.

sympathomimetic	xanthine derivatives
decreased	hypertension
hypotension	increased
intrinsic	mixed
extrinsic	cromolyn
nedocromil	

1. _____ asthma results from a response to an allergen.

2. _____ asthma has both intrinsic and extrinsic factors.

3. _____ asthma results from chronic or recurrent respiratory infections, emotional upset, or exercise.

4. The two major types of bronchodilators are _____ and _____ .

5. Older adults taking sympathomimetic bronchodilators are at a(n) _____ risk for adverse reactions.

6. Effects of oral hypoglycemics or insulin may be _____ when administered with epinephrine.

7. A sympathomimetic drug used concurrently with an oxytocic drug may cause severe _____, and when given with an MAOI may cause severe _____ .

8. Mast cell stabilizers include _____ and _____ .

VIII. LIST

List the requested number of items.

1. List four symptoms of acute bronchospasm that make it a medical emergency.

   a. _____

   b. _____

   c. _____

   d. _____

2. List four conditions in which sympathomimetics are used for treatment.

   a. _____

   b. _____

   c. _____

   d. _____

3. List five conditions in which sympathomimetics are contraindicated.

   a. _____

   b. _____

   c. _____

   d. _____

   e. _____

4. List four adverse reactions of xanthine derivatives.

   a. _____

   b. _____

   c. _____

   d. _____

5. List six signs of theophylline toxicity.

   a. _____

   b. _____

   c. _____

   d. _____

   e. _____

   f. _____

6. List three ways you could suggest to help a patient manage the unpleasant taste of antiasthma drugs.

a. _____

b. _____

c. _____

IX. CLINICAL APPLICATIONS

1. Mr. Y has been prescribed a corticosteroid inhalant for his respiratory disorder. As a healthcare
   worker involved in Mr. Y's care, what might you
   tell Mr. Y about his medication?

2. Mrs. W has been diagnosed with a respiratory
   disorder that requires the regular use of an aerosol inhalant to administer her bronchodilator.
   What should Mrs. W know about the use of this
   medication?

13 Antitussives, Mucolytics, and Expectorants

I. MATCHING

Match the term from Column A with the correct definition from Column B.

COLUMN A

_____ 1. auscultating

_____ 2. mucolytic

_____ 3. nebulization

_____ 4. antitussive

_____ 5. productive cough

COLUMN B

A. A drug used to relieve coughing.
B. The dispersing of a liquid medication in a mist.
C. Listening for sounds within the body.
D. A cough that expels secretions from the lower respiratory tract.
E. A drug that loosens respiratory secretions.

II. MATCHING

Match the generic drug in Column A with the trade name in Column B.

COLUMN A

_____ 1. diphenhydramine HCl

_____ 2. acetylcysteine

_____ 3. dextromethorphan

_____ 4. potassium iodide

_____ 5. dextromethorphan HBr and benzocaine

_____ 6. benzonatate

_____ 7. guaifenesin

COLUMN B

A. Sucrets
B. SSKI
C. Tussin
D. Tessalon Perles
E. Benadryl
F. Spec-T
G. Mucomyst

III. MATCHING

Match the trade name drug in Column A with the type of drug in Column B. You may use an answer more than once.

COLUMN A

_____ 1. Robitussin

_____ 2. Tessalon Perles

_____ 3. Mucomyst

_____ 4. Fenesin

_____ 5. Drixoral Cough

_____ 6. Pima

_____ 7. Benadryl

_____ 8. Vicks Formula 44

_____ 9. Codeine sulfate

COLUMN B

A. Mucolytic
B. Expectorant
C. Narcotic antitussive
D. Nonnarcotic antitussive

IV. TRUE/FALSE

Indicate whether each statement is True (T) or False (F).

_____ 1. To treat the discomfort of upper respiratory tract infections only an antitussive should be used.

_____ 2. A peripherally acting antitussive acts by depressing the cough center located in the medulla.

_____ 3. Antitussives are used to relieve only a nonproductive cough.

_____ 4. A patient with a productive cough should be examined by a healthcare provider before starting any antitussive therapy.

_____ 5. An antitussive that contains an antihistamine may have drowsiness as an adverse reaction.

_____ 6. A mucolytic increases the production of respiratory secretions.

_____ 7. Mucolytics are mainly administered through nebulization.

V. MULTIPLE CHOICE

Circle the letter of the best answer.

1. An example of a centrally acting antitussive is _____ .
   a. benzonatate
   b. potassium iodide
   c. dextromethorphan
   d. guaifenesin
   e. terpin hydrate

2. A peripherally acting antitussive _____ .
   a. acts by anesthetizing stretch receptors in the respiratory passageways
   b. acts by depressing the cough center in the medulla
   c. acts by loosening respiratory secretions
   d. helps to raise thick, tenacious mucus from the respiratory tract
   e. none of the answers are correct

3. Miss T has had a productive cough for 12 days. She has been taking Vicks Formula 44 Cough for 8 days with no relief. What action might you suggest for her?
   a. increase the dose of her current antitussive
   b. buy an antitussive that also contains a mucolytic
   c. change brands of antitussives
   d. consult with her healthcare provider
   e. stop taking all medicines; she is having a rebound reaction to the antitussive

4. A patient with a productive cough who is taking an antitussive may experience _____ .
   a. a pooling of secretions in the lungs
   b. pneumonia and atelectasis
   c. an increased cough reflex
   d. answers a and b are correct
   e. all of the answers are correct

5. Expectorants _____ .
   a. increase the production of respiratory secretions
   b. decrease the viscosity of mucus
   c. help raise secretions from respiratory passages
   d. are used cautiously during pregnancy and lactation
   e. all of the answers are correct

6. When potassium iodide is given as an expectorant to a patient who is also taking a potassium sparing diuretic, what may occur as a result of a drug interaction?
   a. hypokalemia, cardiac arrhythmia, or arrest
   b. hypothyroidism
   c. masking of a medical condition
   d. neither drug will work; they counteract each other
   e. both of the drugs will work better

7. Before a patient is given a mucolytic or an expectorant, he or she must be assessed for _____ .
   a. lung sounds
   b. dyspnea
   c. consistency of sputum
   d. description of sputum
   e. all of the answers are correct

VI. FILL IN THE BLANK

Fill in the blanks using words from the list below.

mucolytic	potassium iodide
additive	dextromethorphan
antitussive	codeine
acetylcysteine	expectorants

1. Using a(n) _____ for a productive cough is often contraindicated.

2. When _____ is administered with MAOIs, patients may experience hypotension, fever, nausea, jerking motions of the leg, or coma.

3. Antitussives containing _____ are classified as Pregnancy Category C drugs.

4. Central nervous system depressants and alcohol may cause _____ depressant effects when administered with antitussives containing codeine.

5. _____ has an additional use in preventing liver damage caused by acetaminophen overdosage.

6. The expectorant _____ is contraindicated during pregnancy.

7. No significant interactions have been reported when _____ are used as directed with the exception of iodine products.

8. _____ drugs can be used as effective adjunctive therapy in cystic fibrosis and in tracheostomy care.

VII. LIST

List the requested number of items.

1. List four conditions in which an antitussive containing codeine is used with caution.

   a. _____

   b. _____

   c. _____

   d. _____

2. List four examples of uses of mucolytics.

   a. _____

   b. _____

   c. _____

   d. _____

VIII. CLINICAL APPLICATIONS

1. Mr. Z is taking an antitussive with codeine at home as part of the treatment of his respiratory disorder. What should Mr. Z and his family be aware of regarding this type of medication?

2. Miss P has been prescribed the expectorant Pima for her respiratory problem. What are the possible adverse reactions with this medication that she should be aware of?

14 Drugs for Heart Conditions: Cardiotonic, Miscellaneous Inotropic, and Antiarrhythmic Drugs

I. MATCHING

Match the term from Column A with the correct definition from Column B.

COLUMN A

_____ 1. atrial fibrillation

_____ 2. arrhythmia

_____ 3. cinchonism

_____ 4. digitalization

_____ 5. ejection fraction

_____ 6. positive inotropic action

_____ 7. proarrhythmic effect

_____ 8. refractory period

COLUMN B

A. The development of a new arrhythmia or the worsening of an existing arrhythmia caused by an antiarrhythmic drug.
B. The amount of blood that the ventricle ejects per beat in relationship to the amount of blood available to eject.
C. A term for quinidine toxicity.
D. A cardiac arrhythmia characterized by rapid contractions of the atrial myocardium, resulting in an irregular and often rapid ventricular rate.
E. The period between transmissions of nerve impulses along a nerve fiber.
F. The increased force of the contraction of the muscle of the heart.
G. A series of doses given until the digitalis drug begins to exert a full therapeutic effect.
H. A disturbance or irregularity in the heart rate or rhythm, or both.

II. MATCHING

Match the generic drug in Column A with the trade name in Column B.

COLUMN A

_____ 1. digoxin immune Fab

_____ 2. flecainide

_____ 3. mexiletine HCl

_____ 4. inamrinone lactate

_____ 5. digoxin

_____ 6. disopyramide

_____ 7. tocainide HCl

_____ 8. esmolol HCl

_____ 9. milrinone lactate

_____ 10. propafenone HCl

_____ 11. acebutolol

_____ 12. procainamide HCl

COLUMN B

A. Primacor
B. Norpace
C. Digitek
D. Sectral
E. Mexitil
F. Rythmol
G. Digibind
H. Tonocard
I. Inocor
J. Brevibloc
K. Tambocor
L. Procanbid

III. MATCHING

Match the Class I drug in Column A with the correct subclass in Column B. You may use an answer more than once.

COLUMN A

_____ 1. propafenone

_____ 2. quinidine

_____ 3. procainamide

_____ 4. mexiletine

_____ 5. flecainide

_____ 6. disopyramide

_____ 7. lidocaine

_____ 8. tocainide

COLUMN B

A. Class IA
B. Class IB
C. Class IC

IV. MATCHING

Match the drug in Column A with the class in Column B. You may use an answer more than once.

COLUMN A

_____ 1. moricizine

_____ 2. milrinone lactate

_____ 3. inamrinone lactate

_____ 4. mexiletine HCl

_____ 5. disopyramide

_____ 6. digoxin

_____ 7. tocainide HCl

_____ 8. procainamide HCl

_____ 9. verapamil

_____ 10. amiodarone

COLUMN B

A. Cardiotonic
B. Antiarrhythmic

V. MATCHING

Match the drug in Column A with the class in Column B. You may use an answer more than once.

_____ 1. lidocaine HCL

_____ 2. moricizine

_____ 3. acebutolol

_____ 4. quinidine sulfate

_____ 5. esmolol HCl

_____ 6. quinidine HCl

_____ 7. propafenone HCl

_____ 8. flecainide

_____ 9. bretylium

_____ 10. ibutilide

_____ 11. amiodarone

_____ 12. verapamil

_____ 13. diltiazem

_____ 14. dofetilide

COLUMN B

A. Class I
B. Class II
C. Class III
D. Class IV

VI. MATCHING

Indicate whether the drug in Column A would cause an increase or a decrease in the digitalis plasma level of a patient. You may use an answer more than once.

COLUMN A

_____ 1. aminoglycosides

_____ 2. macrolides

_____ 3. benzodiazepines

_____ 4. antacids

_____ 5. quinidine

_____ 6. St. John's wort

_____ 7. activated charcoal

_____ 8. tetracycline

COLUMN B

A. Increase in digitalis plasma level
B. Decrease in digitalis plasma level

VII. TRUE/FALSE

Indicate whether each statement is True (T) or False (F).

_____ 1. Cardiotonics are used to improve the efficiency and contraction of the heart muscle.

_____ 2. The goal of antiarrhythmic drug therapy is to inhibit normal cardiac function and to prevent a life-threatening cardiac rhythm.

_____ 3. Digitalis glycosides are another term for a cardiotonic.

_____ 4. Positive inotropic action results in increased cardiac output and decreased heart rate.

_____ 5. Normal doses of a cardiotonic drug may cause toxic drug effects.

_____ 6. Hypokalemia is a concern for patients receiving digoxin immune Fab.

_____ 7. Fetal toxicity and neonatal death have resulted from maternal digoxin overdosage.

_____ 8. A patient receiving a miscellaneous inotropic drug must have continuous cardiac monitoring.

_____ 9. Renal function in patients taking cardiotonics is not a consideration since the drug is metabolized by the liver.

_____ 10. Lidocaine works by reducing the number of stimuli that can pass along myocardial fibers, which decreases the pulse rate and corrects the arrhythmia.

_____ 11. Ibutilide and dofetilide are used to convert atrial fibrillation or atrial flutter back to sinus rhythm.

_____ 12. Class IV antiarrhythmic drugs are also called calcium antagonists.

_____ 13. Antiarrhythmics may sometimes be used to treat migraine headaches.

_____ 14. Antiarrhythmic drugs never cause new arrhythmias.

_____ 15. Proarrhythmic effects of a drug are easy to distinguish from a pre-existing arrhythmia.

_____ 16. Lidocaine is generally reserved for the treatment of life-threatening ventricular arrhythmias.

VIII. MULTIPLE CHOICE

Circle the letter of the best answer.

1. The most commonly used cardiotonic drug is _____
   a. lidocaine HCl
   b. digoxin
   c. tocainide HCl
   d. esmolol HCl
   e. acebutolol

2. Cardiotonics are used to treat _____ .
   a. heart failure
   b. ventricular fibrillation
   c. atrial fibrillation
   d. answers a and b are correct
   e. answers a and c are correct

3. Mrs. Q is receiving digitalis for her heart failure. If she would mention _____, the healthcare worker should notify the healthcare provider immediately.
   a. blurred vision
   b. anorexia
   c. headache
   d. abnormal heart beat
   e. all of the answers are correct

4. Which of the following drugs is used more often in the short-term management of severe heart failure that is not controlled by digitalis?
   a. digoxin immune fab
   b. milrinone
   c. esmolol
   d. thiazide
   e. inamrinone

5. Miscellaneous inotropic drugs such as inamrinone or milrinone _____ .
   a. cure heart failure
   b. help manage arrhythmias
   c. control the signs and symptoms of heart failure
   d. decrease cardiac output
   e. prevent right-sided ventricular failure

6. Mr. T was accidentally given a double dose of digoxin at the hospital. To treat this potentially life-threatening toxicity, the healthcare provider may need to _____ .

   a. withdraw the drug from his next scheduled treatment regimen
   b. change his medicine
   c. order digoxin immune Fab
   d. answers a and c are correct
   e. answers a and b are correct

7. Digitalization of a patient _____ .

   a. involves a series of doses
   b. includes a first dose of approximately half the total dose
   c. may involve injections or tablets
   d. answers a and b are correct
   e. answers a, b, and c are correct

8. It is important that family members and patients undergoing long-term cardiotonic therapy _____ .

   a. understand the need to take the drug as prescribed
   b. take their pulse as directed
   c. are aware of drug interactions
   d. follow dietary recommendations
   e. all of the answers are correct

9. Antiarrhythmic drugs are classified _____ .

   a. according to their effects on the action potential of cardiac cells
   b. according to their presumed mechanism of action
   c. based on their chemical components
   d. based on their effects on the muscular tissue of the heart
   e. answers a and b are correct

10. Which class of antiarrhythmic drug has a membrane-stabilizing effect on the cells of the myocardium?

    a. Class I
    b. Class II
    c. Class III
    d. Class IV
    e. none of the answers are correct.

11. An example of an antiarrhythmic that acts by decreasing the rate of diastolic depolarization in the ventricles and increases the fiber threshold is _____ .

    a. disopyramide
    b. quinidine
    c. procainamide

    d. lidocaine
    e. verapamil

12. Which of the following drugs works by raising the threshold of the ventricular myocardium?

    a. quinidine
    b. procainamide
    c. verapamil
    d. lidocaine
    e. esmolol

13. Which class of antiarrhythmic acts by having a direct stabilizing action on the myocardium?

    a. Class IA
    b. Class IB
    c. Class IC
    d. Class II
    e. Class III

14. Class II antiarrhythmic drugs work by _____ .

    a. shortening the refractory period
    b. blocking stimulation of beta receptors of the heart
    c. stimulating alpha receptors
    d. shortening repolarization
    e. decreasing the threshold

15. Which of the Class III antiarrhythmic drugs selectively blocks potassium channels?

    a. ibutilide
    b. dofetilide
    c. bretylium
    d. amiodarone
    e. none of the answers are correct

16. Older adults taking antiarrhythmics are at increased risk for _____ .

    a. proarrhythmias
    b. worsening of existing arrhythmias
    c. hypotension
    d. congestive heart failure
    e. all of the answers are correct

17. Cinchonism may be indicated by all of the following symptoms except _____ .

    a. tinnitus and vertigo
    b. increased sensitivity to noises
    c. headache and light-headedness
    d. nausea
    e. all of the answers are correct

18. Miss B is taking procainamide and is experiencing nausea and vomiting. As her healthcare worker, what might you suggest to her to help deal with this adverse reaction?

    a. Eat only three large meals.
    b. Smoking may ease the discomfort.

c. Split the doses into several smaller ones.
d. Try eating smaller more frequent meals.
e. Chewing the tablets will help with the discomfort.

19. An adverse reaction of disopyramide is urinary retention. This is caused by _____ .

   a. beta-adrenergic stimulation
   b. anticholinergic effects
   c. cholinergic blocking effects
   d. beta-adrenergic blocking effects
   e. none of the answers are correct

20. Dofetilide is not given with cimetidine because _____ .

   a. dofetilide levels may increase by 50%
   b. cimetidine levels may increase by 50%
   c. dofetilide levels may decrease by 50%
   d. cimetidine levels may decrease by 50%
   e. answers a and b are correct

IX. RECALL FACTS

Indicate which of the following statements are Facts with an F. If the statement is not a fact, leave the line blank.

About Patient Assessment Before Cardiotonic Therapy

_____ 1. Blood pressure, pulse, and respiratory rate

_____ 2. Lung sounds and appearance of sputum

_____ 3. Height and sex of patient

_____ 4. Weight

_____ 5. Presence of edema

_____ 6. Jugular vein distention

_____ 7. Environment patient works in

_____ 8. Availability of medical care

About Patient Assessment Before Antiarrhythmic Therapy

_____ 1. Blood pressure, pulse, and respiratory rate

_____ 2. Weight

_____ 3. Urinary output

_____ 4. Cardiac monitoring available

_____ 5. ECG

_____ 6. Lab tests

X. FILL IN THE BLANK

Fill in the blanks using words from the list below.

additive	hypokalemia
hypomagnesemia	slowed
same	decreased
rapid	beta blocker
short	ACE inhibitors
diuretics	gradual
lidocaine	propranolol
rapid	

1. The first three lines of treatment for heart failure are _____, _____, and _____.

2. Digoxin has a(n) _____ onset and a(n) _____ duration of action.

3. When a cardiotonic is taken with food, absorption is _____ but the amount of drug absorbed is the _____, unless it is taken with a high-fiber meal; then absorption may be _____.

4. Two methods of digitalization may be used when a patient starts treatment with a cardiotonic: the _____ method or the _____ method.

5. Patients receiving a cardiotonic drug and a diuretic are at risk for _____ and _____.

6. Patients taking _____ or _____ require constant cardiac monitoring.

7. When two antiarrhythmic drugs are given concurrently, the patient may experience _____ effects.

XI. LIST

List the requested number of items.

1. List the two ways in which cardiotonics act.

   a. _____

   b. _____

2. List the four factors that influence the dose of cardiotonics that a patient may receive.

a. _____

b. _____

c. _____

d. _____

3. List the four systems that may show signs of digitalis toxicity.

a. _____

b. _____

c. _____

d. _____

4. List four conditions in which a cardiotonic is contraindicated.

a. _____

b. _____

c. _____

d. _____

5. List four arrhythmic conditions in which antiarrhythmic drugs could be used.

a. _____

b. _____

c. _____

d. _____

6. List three times when a proarrhythmic effect is more likely to occur.

a. _____

b. _____

c. _____

7. List five antiarrhythmic drugs that may cause agranulocytosis.

a. _____

b. _____

c. _____

d. _____

e. _____

8. List four conditions in which antiarrhythmic drugs are contraindicated.

a. _____

b. _____

c. _____

d. _____

XII. CLINICAL APPLICATIONS

1. Mrs. K will be continuing her cardiotonic drug therapy at home after her discharge. As the healthcare worker assigned to her discharge, what important points should you make sure she understands about this type of medication?

2. You suspect that Mr. Q has right-sided ventricular heart failure. What symptoms would you expect to observe in Mr. Q as his disease progresses?

Antianginal and Peripheral Vasodilating Drugs

I. MATCHING

Match the term from Column A with the correct definition from Column B.

COLUMN A

_____ 1. angina

_____ 2. intermittent claudication

_____ 3. lumen

_____ 4. prophylaxis

_____ 5. transdermal system

COLUMN B

A. A group of symptoms characterized by pain in the calf muscle of one or both legs.
B. Prevention.
C. A convenient form of drug administration in which the drug is impregnated in a pad and absorbed through the skin.
D. A disorder that causes decreased oxygen supply to the heart muscle and results in chest pain or pressure.
E. The inside diameter of a vessel.

II. MATCHING

Match the generic nitroglycerin drugs in Column A with the trade name in Column B.

COLUMN A

_____ 1. nitroglycerin intravenous

_____ 2. nitroglycerin translingual

_____ 3. nitroglycerin transmucosal

_____ 4. nitroglycerin sublingual

_____ 5. nitroglycerin sustained release

_____ 6. nitroglycerin topical

_____ 7. nitroglycerin transdermal system

COLUMN B

A. Nitroglyn
B. NitroQuick
C. Nitro-Bid
D. Nitro-Bid IV
E. Deponit
F. Nitrogard
G. Nitrolingual

III. MATCHING

Match the generic calcium channel blocker in Column A with the trade name in Column B.

COLUMN A

_____ 1. diltiazem HCl

_____ 2. nicardipine HCl

_____ 3. nifedipine

_____ 4. verapamil

_____ 5. bepridil HCl

_____ 6. amlodipine

COLUMN B

A. Cardizem
B. Calan
C. Cardene
D. Vascor
E. Procardia
F. Norvasc

IV. MATCHING

Match the antianginal or peripheral vasodilating generic drug in Column A with the trade name in Column B.

COLUMN A

_____ 1. cilostazol

_____ 2. isosorbide mononitrate, oral

_____ 3. isoxsuprine HCl

_____ 4. isosorbide dinitrate, oral

_____ 5. papaverine HCl

_____ 6. isosorbide dinitrate, sublingual

_____ 7. amyl nitrite

COLUMN B

A. amyl nitrite
B. Isordil
C. Dilatrate-SR
D. ISMO, Imdur
E. Pletal
F. Vasodilan
G. Pavabid Plateau

V. TRUE/FALSE

Indicate whether each statement is True (T) or False (F).

_____ 1. Antianginal drugs work by causing peripheral vasodilation.

_____ 2. Nitrate drugs work by having a direct relaxing effect on the smooth muscle layer of blood vessels.

_____ 3. Nitrates are used to treat angina pectoris.

_____ 4. Oral nitroglycerin may be swallowed without regard to meals.

_____ 5. Patients using nitroglycerin for long-term treatment can develop a tolerance to the drug.

_____ 6. The effect of calcium channel blockers is the same as the effect of nitrates.

_____ 7. Adverse reactions to calcium channel blockers are frequently severe and often require discontinuation of the drug.

_____ 8. Rebound angina is probably caused by an increase in calcium ions flowing into cells causing coronary artery spasm.

_____ 9. Patients taking calcium channel blockers should be watched for signs of congestive heart failure.

_____ 10. Peripheral vasodilating drugs show conclusively that they increase blood flow to ischemic areas of the body.

_____ 11. Patients taking peripheral vasodilating drugs may see no significant improvement for several weeks after therapy is begun.

_____ 12. L-arginine appears to work by increasing nitric acid concentrations.

VI. MULTIPLE CHOICE

Circle the letter of the best answer.

1. Which of the following drugs is used to treat Raynaud's disease?
   a. cilostazol
   b. isoxsuprine HCl
   c. nifedipine
   d. papaverine
   e. diltiazem HCl

2. Peripheral vasodilating drugs act to _____ .
   a. inhibit platelet aggregation
   b. relieve the pain of angina
   c. increase calcium ion concentration in the cells
   d. reduce inflammation
   e. block alpha-adrenergic nerves and stimulate beta-adrenergic nerves

3. Pletal has a generic name of _____ .
   a. cilostazol
   b. isoxsuprine HCl
   c. papaverine HCl
   d. verapamil HCl
   e. amyl nitrate

4. Because of the action of peripheral vasodilating drugs, which adverse reaction might you anticipate in a patient?
   a. dysuria
   b. hypertension
   c. hypotension
   d. dry mouth
   e. paleness

5. Mrs. C has been taking a peripheral vasodilating drug regularly for several weeks for a peripheral vascular disorder. What signs might Mrs. C begin to note that would indicate an improvement in her condition?
   a. a decrease in pain
   b. an increase in warmth of extremities
   c. a stronger peripheral pulse
   d. changes in the color of her extremities
   e. all of the answers are correct

6. L-arginine should be used with caution by patients who have _____ .
   a. congestive heart failure
   b. hypertension
   c. angina
   d. sickle cell anemia
   e. been taking MAOIs

7. Mr. V has called the office and said that his episode of chest pain has not responded to three doses of nitroglycerin given every 5 minutes for 15 minutes. What might you tell him to do?

   a. Take another dose and call back in 15 minutes.
   b. Increase the dose and try it three more times in 15 minutes.
   c. Try chewing the tablets instead of placing them under the tongue.
   d. Notify his healthcare provider immediately.
   e. None of the answers are correct.

8. Antianginal drugs include the _____ .

   a. phosphodiesterase II inhibitors
   b. nitrates
   c. adrenergic blocking agents
   d. calcium channel blockers
   e. answers b and d are correct

9. Nitrates _____ .

   a. increase the lumen of the artery
   b. increase the volume of blood flow
   c. increase the oxygen supply to the cardiac tissue
   d. decrease chest pain or pressure
   e. all of the answers are correct

10. A common adverse reaction of nitrate administration is _____ .

    a. vomiting
    b. headaches
    c. diarrhea
    d. dry mouth
    e. CNS stimulation

11. In which of the following conditions are the nitrates contraindicated?

    a. renal failure
    b. closed-angle glaucoma
    c. cirrhosis
    d. leukemia
    e. orthostatic hypotension

12. The transdermal system of nitroglycerin administration has better results when the patient _____ .

    a. applies the patch at the same location repeatedly
    b. leaves the patch on for 10 to 12 hours and then removes the patch for 10 to 12 hours
    c. rubs the patch on the skin
    d. places the patch on a mucous membrane
    e. wets the patch before application

13. Calcium channel blockers are used to _____ .

    a. prevent anginal pain
    b. treat vasospastic angina
    c. treat chronic stable angina
    d. stop anginal pain once started
    e. answers a, b, and c are correct

14. Mr. F is an 85 year-old man taking an antianginal drug. What should his healthcare provider watch for to minimize his risk of injury?

    a. dry mouth
    b. increased postural hypotension
    c. peripheral edema
    d. skin rash
    e. dermatitis

15. Discontinuation of a calcium channel blocker _____ .

    a. may cause an increase in chest pain
    b. should be done gradually
    c. may cause rebound angina
    d. may cause coronary arteries to spasm
    e. all of the answers are correct

VII. RECALL FACTS

Indicate which of the following statements are Facts with an F. If the statement is not a fact, leave the line blank.

About Contraindications, Precautions, and Interactions of Calcium Channel Blockers

_____ 1. They are contraindicated in pregnancy and during lactation.

_____ 2. They are contraindicated in patients who have sick sinus syndrome.

_____ 3. They are contraindicated in patients with second- or third-degree AV block.

_____ 4. Effects are decreased when given with cimetidine or ranitidine.

_____ 5. They have an antiplatelet effect when given with aspirin.

_____ 6. They may increase a patient's risk for digitalis toxicity when give with digoxin.

About Patient Management Issues with Nitrates

_____ 1. With treatment, angina should decrease in frequency or be eliminated.

_____ 2. A dry mouth will decrease the absorption of sublingual or buccal forms of the drug.

_____ 3. They may be administered in a topical form.

_____ 4. Patients never develop a tolerance to nitroglycerin.

_____ 5. Oral nitroglycerin should be taken on an empty stomach.

VIII. FILL IN THE BLANK

Fill in the blanks using words from the list below.

hypotensive	disappear
increased	decreased
Isordil	increased
decreased	Nitrostat
intermittent	pulse rate
claudication	
gradual	

1. _____ is used for prevention and long-term treatment of angina, whereas _____ is used to relieve the pain of acute anginal attacks.

2. A(n) _____ hypotensive effect may be seen when nitrates are administered with antihypertensives or alcohol, whereas a(n) _____ effect of heparin may be exhibited if IV nitroglycerin is administered.

3. The effects of calcium channel blockers are _____ when given with cimetidine or ranitidine, but are _____ when given with phenobarbital or phenytoin.

4. Older adults may have a greater _____ effect while taking antianginal drugs than younger adults.

5. Most adverse reactions of antianginal drugs will _____ after a period of time.

6. A manifestation of peripheral vascular disease in which other atherosclerotic lesions develop in the leg and cause pain in the calf may lead to _____.

7. Peripheral vasodilating drugs can cause a physiological increase in the _____.

8. Improvement will be _____ in the treatment of peripheral vascular disease.

IX. LIST

List the requested number of items.

1. List four forms of administration of nitrates.

   a. _____

   b. _____

   c. _____

   d. _____

2. List four common adverse reactions to calcium channel blockers.

   a. _____

   b. _____

   c. _____

   d. _____

3. List three disorders in which a peripheral vasodilating drug may be used.

   a. _____

   b. _____

   c. _____

4. List the significant drug-drug interactions associated with peripheral vasodilating drugs administration.

   a. _____

   b. _____

   c. _____

5. List four conditions that the herbal supplement L-arginine is marketed to improve or prevent.

a. _____

b. _____

c. _____

d. _____

X. CLINICAL APPLICATIONS

1. Mr. B is taking a vasodilating drug. Give Mr. B a short explanation about how these drugs may work to relieve some or all of his symptoms.

2. Explain to Miss T how to administer her sublingual or buccal nitrate medication.

16 Antihypertensive Drugs

I. MATCHING

Match the term from Column A with the correct definition from Column B.

COLUMN A

_____ 1. aldosterone

_____ 2. endogenous

_____ 3. hypertension

_____ 4. isolated systolic hypertension

_____ 5. malignant hypertension

_____ 6. secondary hypertension

COLUMN B

A. A condition of only an elevated systolic pressure.
B. A systolic pressure greater than 140 mm Hg and a diastolic pressure greater than 90 mm Hg.
C. Hypertension in which a direct cause can be identified.
D. A hormone that promotes the retention of sodium and water, which may contribute to a rise in blood pressure.
E. Hypertension in which the diastolic pressure usually exceeds 130 mm Hg.
F. Substances normally manufactured by the body.

II. MATCHING

Match the ACE inhibitor or angiotensin receptor antagonist generic drug in Column A with the trade name in Column B.

COLUMN A

_____ 1. irbesartan

_____ 2. ramipril

_____ 3. fosinopril sodium

_____ 4. losartan potassium

_____ 5. valsartan

_____ 6. captopril

_____ 7. benazepril HCl

_____ 8. quinapril HCl

_____ 9. moexipril HCl

_____ 10. enalapril

COLUMN B

A. Monopril
B. Diovan
C. Capoten
D. Avapro
E. Cozaar
F. Lotensin
G. Altace
H. Vasotec
I. Accupril
J. Univasc

III. MATCHING

Match the drug in Column A with the type of drug in Column B. You may use an answer more than once.

COLUMN A

_____ 1. enalapril

_____ 2. perindopril erbumine

_____ 3. eprosartan mesylate

_____ 4. irbesartan

_____ 5. telmisartan

_____ 6. benazepril HCl

_____ 7. lisinopril

_____ 8. candesartan cilexetil

COLUMN B

A. ACE inhibitor
B. Angiotensin II receptor antagonist

IV. MATCHING

Match the generic antihypertensive drug in Column A with the trade name in Column B.

COLUMN A

_____ 1. penbutolol sulfate

_____ 2. nadolol

_____ 3. pindolol

_____ 4. guanfacine HCl

_____ 5. carvedilol

_____ 6. clonidine HCl

_____ 7. guanadrel

_____ 8. mecamylamine HCl

_____ 9. atenolol

_____ 10. guanethidine monosulfate

_____ 11. minoxidil

_____ 12. doxazosin mesylate

COLUMN B

A. Tenex
B. Coreg
C. Catapres
D. Levatol
E. Hylorel
F. Corgard
G. Ismelin
H. Visken
 I. Cardura
 J. Tenormin
K. Loniten
L. Inversine

V. MATCHING

Match the generic antihypertensive drug in Column A with the type of antihypertensive in Column B. You may use an answer more than once.

COLUMN A

_____ 1. reserpine

_____ 2. propranolol HCl

_____ 3. prazosin

_____ 4. nadolol

_____ 5. guanabenz acetate

_____ 6. guanadrel

_____ 7. hydralazine HCl

_____ 8. terazosin

_____ 9. acebutolol HCl

_____ 10. methyldopa

_____ 11. bisoprolol fumarate

_____ 12. guanfacine HCl

COLUMN B

A. Peripheral vasodilator
B. Beta-adrenergic blocking drug
C. Antiadrenergic—centrally acting
D. Antiadrenergic—peripherally acting
E. Alpha-adrenergic blocking drug

VI. TRUE/FALSE

Indicate whether each statement is True (T) or False (F).

_____ 1. With proper treatment essential hypertension can be cured.

_____ 2. Diuretics and beta-blocking drugs may sometimes be prescribed first for the treatment of hypertension.

_____ 3. Treatment of hypertension often involves changing medications or adding a second drug to the therapy regimen.

_____ 4. All antihypertensive drugs work equally well, so treatment plans are easy to establish.

_____ 5. When monitoring the blood pressure of a patient receiving antihypertensive therapy, it does not matter whether the person is always in the same position.

_____ 6. Hypertension only occurs in older adults.

_____ 7. Older adults should be given a lower dose of nitroprusside because they seem to be more sensitive to its hypotensive effects.

VII. MULTIPLE CHOICE

Circle the letter of the best answer.

1. Which of the types of drugs listed below can be used to treat hypertension?
   a. calcium channel blockers
   b. antiadrenergic drugs
   c. ACE inhibitors
   d. diuretics
   e. all of the answers are correct

2. ACE inhibitors lower blood pressure by _____ .
   a. preventing the conversion of angiotensin I to angiotensin II
   b. preventing sodium and water retention
   c. blocking receptor sites for angiotensin II

d. answers a and b are correct

e. answers a, b, and c are correct

3. Antihypertensive drugs _____ .

   a. are used to treat hypertension

   b. may cause postural or orthostatic hypotension

   c. must be discontinued gradually over 2 to 4 days

   d. may cause the patient to become dehydrated and alter the electrolyte balance

   e. all of the answers are correct

4. Mr. G is being treated with a diuretic for his hypertension. What signs or symptoms should a healthcare worker be alert for?

   a. hyponatremia

   b. dehydration

   c. hypokalemia

   d. electrolyte imbalance

   e. all of the answers are correct

5. Which type of antihypertensive drug is a Pregnancy Category D during the second and third trimesters and therefore is contraindicated?

   a. angiotensin II receptor antagonists

   b. ACE inhibitors

   c. peripheral vasodilators

   d. antiadrenergics-centrally acting

   e. α-adrenergic blocking drugs

6. From which of the herbal remedies or supplements listed below has it been demonstrated that hypertensive patients may benefit?

   a. hawthorn extracts

   b. calcium and magnesium

   c. vitamin E and aspirin

   d. garlic and onion

   e. ginkgo biloba

7. Mr. S is being treated for hypertension. His healthcare worker notes that after weighing him he has gained 3 pounds since the previous day. The healthcare worker should _____ .

   a. keep Mr. S from drinking water

   b. report this information to the healthcare provider

   c. encourage Mr. S to stay with his diet

   d. ignore the information as he was wearing his shoes on the scale

   e. not worry unless his blood pressure is also higher

VIII. RECALL FACTS

Indicate which of the following statements are Facts with an F. If the statement is not a fact, leave the line blank.

About Life Style Changes That Reduce the Risk of Hypertension

_____ 1. Weight loss

_____ 2. Quit smoking

_____ 3. Increase fluid intake

_____ 4. Eliminate carbohydrates from diet

_____ 5. Reduce stress

_____ 6. Increase salt consumption

_____ 7. Regular aerobic exercise

_____ 8. Diet changes such as a DASH diet

_____ 9. Move to a warm, dry climate

_____ 10. Use an electric blanket

About Increased Effects of Antihypertensives, ACE Inhibitors, or Angiotensin II Receptor Antagonists

_____ 1. When administered with another antihypertensive

_____ 2. When administered with a diuretic

_____ 3. When administered with an MAOI

_____ 4. When administered with NSAID

_____ 5. When administered with antacids

_____ 6. When administered with phenobarbital

IX. FILL IN THE BLANK

Fill in the blanks using words from the list below.

organ damage	sodium
gradually	high
doxazosin mesylate	metoprolol
atenolol	timolol maleate
nadolol	propanolol HCl
lifetime	lumen
diazoxide	nitroprusside

1. Once essential hypertension develops, management of this disorder is a _____ task.

2. Patients with malignant hypertension experience _____ as a result of hypertension.

3. Vasodilation increases the _____ of the arterial blood vessel.

4. Diuretics increase the excretion of _____ from the body.

5. _____ and _____ are IV drugs that can be used to treat hypertensive emergencies.

6. When discontinuing an antihypertensive drug, the dosage is _____ reduced over 2 to 4 days.

7. It has been suggested that blood pressure can be lowered by a diet _____ in magnesium, calcium, and potassium.

8. _____, _____, and _____ can be used to treat angina pectoris.

9. _____ can be used to treat benign prostatic hypertrophy.

10. _____ and _____ are sometimes used to treat migraines.

X. LIST

List the requested number of items.

1. List four risk factors for hypertension.
   a. _____
   b. _____
   c. _____
   d. _____

2. List four things you could advise a patient to do to minimize their risk of injury from postural hypotension.
   a. _____
   b. _____
   c. _____
   d. _____

3. List six types of drugs used to treat hypertension.
   a. _____
   b. _____
   c. _____
   d. _____
   e. _____
   f. _____

4. List four antihypertensive drugs with vasodilating activity.
   a. _____
   b. _____
   c. _____
   d. _____

5. List three antihypertensive drugs used to treat glaucoma.
   a. _____
   b. _____
   c. _____

XI. CLINICAL APPLICATIONS

1. Mr. E is taking multiple drugs to treat his hypertension. His risk for orthostatic hypotension is increased because of this. What are several things that Mr. E could do to help reduce his risk of injury?

2. Mrs. P has been taking two different antihypertensive medications over the past several months, but her blood pressure still remains elevated. What might the healthcare provider try next to bring Mrs. P's blood pressure down?

17 Antihyperlipidemic Drugs

I. MATCHING

Match the term from Column A with the correct definition from Column B.

COLUMN A

_____ 1. atherosclerosis

_____ 2. catalyst

_____ 3. cholesterol

_____ 4. HDL

_____ 5. lipids

_____ 6. lipoprotein

_____ 7. LDL

_____ 8. triglycerides

COLUMN B

A. One of the lipids in the blood.
B. A substance that accelerates a chemical reaction without itself undergoing a change.
C. Fats or fat-like substances in the blood.
D. Transports cholesterol to peripheral cells.
E. A disorder in which lipid deposits accumulate on the lining of the blood vessels, eventually producing degenerative changes and obstruction of blood flow.
F. A type of lipid in the blood.
G. A lipid-containing protein
H. Carry cholesterol from peripheral cells to the liver

II. MATCHING

Match the generic drug in Column A with the trade name in Column B.

COLUMN A

_____ 1. cholestyramine

_____ 2. atorvastatin

_____ 3. lovastatin

_____ 4. clofibrate

_____ 5. simvastatin

_____ 6. niacin

_____ 7. fenofibrate

_____ 8. colestipol HCl

_____ 9. fluvastatin

_____ 10. pravastatin

COLUMN B

A. Zocor
B. Lipitor
C. Mevacor
D. LoCHOLEST
E. Atromid-S
F. Tricor
G. Lescol
H. Niaspan
I. Pravachol
J. Colestid

III. MATCHING

Match the drug in Column A with the type of antihyperlipidemic in Column B. You may use an answer more than once.

COLUMN A

_____ 1. colesevelam HCl

_____ 2. atorvastatin

_____ 3. lovastatin

_____ 4. clofibrate

_____ 5. gemfibrozil

_____ 6. cholestyramine

_____ 7. simvastatin

_____ 8. fluvastatin

_____ 9. pravastatin

_____ 10. fenofibrate

_____ 11. colestipol HCl

COLUMN B

A. Fibric acid derivatives
B. HMG-CoA reductase inhibitors
C. Bile acid sequestrants

IV. MATCHING

Match the fibric acid derivative drug in Column A with the correct action in Column B.

COLUMN A

_____ 1. clofibrate

_____ 2. fenofibrate

_____ 3. gemfibrozil

COLUMN B

A. Increases the excretion of cholesterol in the feces and decreased triglyceride production by the liver
B. Stimulates the breakdown of VLDL to LDL
C. Reduces VLDL and stimulates catabolism of triglyceride-rich lipoproteins

V. TRUE/FALSE

Indicate whether each statement is True (T) or False (F).

_____ 1. The two lipids found in blood are cholesterol and triglycerides.

_____ 2. Lipoproteins can bind water-insoluble lipids and transport them throughout the body.

_____ 3. When the cells of the body have the cholesterol that they need, they discard the excess into the blood where it can then form atherosclerotic plaque.

_____ 4. High-density lipoprotein is considered to be the "good" lipoprotein and should be a high number.

_____ 5. In general, the higher one's LDL level, the greater the risk for heart disease.

_____ 6. Bile acid sequestrants work by binding bile acids to form an insoluble substance that is excreted in the feces, causing the liver to use cholesterol to make more bile.

_____ 7. HMG-CoA reductase inhibitors are used to treat high serum triglyceride levels when diet alone has not lowered the level.

_____ 8. All fibric acid derivatives work in the same way.

_____ 9. The fibric acid derivatives may trigger the formation of gallstones or cholecystitis.

_____ 10. Niacin is used to help lower serum cholesterol levels.

VI. MULTIPLE CHOICE

Circle the letter of the best answer.

1. The target LDL level for treatment is _____ .
   a. less than 130 mg/dL
   b. greater than 40 mg/dL
   c. between 150 and 200 mg/dL
   d. equal to the cholesterol level
   e. none of the answers are correct

2. Mr. H has had no decrease in his cholesterol level with a diet and exercise program. Which of the three types of antihyperlipidemic drugs might the healthcare provider recommend?
   a. niacin
   b. fibric acid derivatives
   c. HMG-CoA reductase inhibitors
   d. bile acid sequestrants
   e. none of these drugs will help Mr. C lower his cholesterol

3. Bile acid sequestrants _____ .
   a. should be administered alone
   b. decrease the absorption of other drugs
   c. are contraindicated in complete biliary obstruction
   d. may increase the risk of bleeding when given with oral anticoagulants
   e. all of the answers are correct

4. _____ appears to inhibit the manufacture of cholesterol or promote the breakdown of cholesterol.
   a. Niacin
   b. Bile acid sequestrants
   c. HMG-CoA reductase inhibitors
   d. Fibric acid derivatives
   e. All of the answers are correct

5. Mrs. S is being treated with pravastatin. At her regular check-up she reports that she has just started to note some muscle pain and has had a low-grade fever. As part of her healthcare team, you tell her _____ .
   a. she probably has a touch of the flu
   b. it is a common adverse reaction of her medicine

c. it will go away as she gets used to the medicine

d. that you will report this to her healthcare provider immediately

e. it means that the medication is working

6. Which fibric acid derivative is not thought to be effective for the prevention of coronary heart disease?

a. clofibrate

b. gemfibrozil

c. fenofibrate

d. niacin

e. both answers a and b

7. Mrs. L wants to know why so many people take garlic as a dietary supplement to help their cardiovascular system. As a healthcare worker you can explain to her that garlic _____ .

a. helps to lower serum cholesterol and triglyceride levels

b. improves the HDL to LDL ratio

c. lowers blood pressure

d. helps prevent atherosclerosis

e. all of the answers are correct

8. Ms. M has been faithfully taking her antihyperlipidemic drug for almost 4 months with no improvement in her blood cholesterol levels. What treatment options are left for her with medications?

a. She should continue with the same therapy for 3 more months.

b. Her drug regimen may need to be modified.

c. She should discontinue all of her drugs because they obviously are not working.

d. She may need multiple medications.

e. She may need higher doses of her current drug.

VII. RECALL FACTS

Indicate which of the following statements are Facts with an F. If the statement is not a fact, leave the line blank.

About Bile Acid Sequestrant Administration

_____ 1. Should be taken before meals unless instructed otherwise.

_____ 2. Cholestyramine powder can be placed safely on the tongue.

_____ 3. Colestipol granules do not dissolve, so the preparation must be stirred until it is ready to drink.

_____ 4. Colesevelam tablets can be taken without regard for meals.

_____ 5. It is uncommon to experience constipation, flatulence, nausea, or heartburn after administration of bile acid sequestrants.

About Risk Factors for Developing Hyperlipidemia

_____ 1. Cigarette smoking

_____ 2. Hypertension

_____ 3. Obesity

_____ 4. Anemia

_____ 5. Diabetes

_____ 6. Age

VIII. FILL IN THE BLANK

Fill in the blanks using words from the list below.

LDLs	garlic
niacin	constipation
HDLs	240
150	rhabdomyolysis

1. A cholesterol level greater than _____ mg/dL and a triglyceride level greater than _____ mg/dL could contribute to atherosclerosis.

2. _____ transport cholesterol to peripheral cells while _____ carry cholesterol from the peripheral cells to the liver to be metabolized.

3. A common adverse reaction of bile acid sequestrants is _____ .

4. _____ is a rare but serious adverse reaction of HMG-CoA reductase inhibitors.

5. Some adverse reactions of _____ include flushing of the skin, a sensation of warmth, and severe itching or tingling.

6. _____ is excreted in breast milk and may cause colic in infants.

IX. LIST

List the requested number of items.

1. List four factors that contribute to hyperlipidemia.

   a. _____

   b. _____

   c. _____

   d. _____

2. List four therapeutic life changes that can help lower a patient's cholesterol level.

   a. _____

   b. _____

   c. _____

   d. _____

3. List four things that a patient may do to lessen constipation that results from bile acid sequestrant use.

   a. _____

   b. _____

   c. _____

   d. _____

4. List the two types of antihyperlipidemic drugs that may lead to rhabdomyolysis.

   a. _____

   b. _____

5. List four things that a healthcare provider should do when dealing with a patient using diet and drugs to control high blood cholesterol levels.

   a. _____

   b. _____

   c. _____

   d. _____

X. CLINICAL APPLICATION

1. Mrs. Z is taking a bile acid sequestrant to help lower her serum cholesterol level. What adverse reactions might she expect while taking this medication?

18 Anticoagulant, Thrombolytic, and Anti-Anemia Drugs

I. MATCHING

Match the term from Column A with the correct definition from Column B.

COLUMN A

_____ 1. fibrolytic drugs

_____ 2. hemostasis

_____ 3. prothrombin

_____ 4. thrombolytic drugs

_____ 5. thrombosis

_____ 6. thrombus

COLUMN B

A. The formation of a clot.
B. Blood clot.
C. Drugs designed to dissolve existing clots.
D. A substance that is essential for the clotting of blood.
E. A process that stops bleeding in a blood vessel.
F. Another name for thrombolytic drugs.

II. MATCHING

Match the generic drug name in Column A with the type of anemia it is used to treat in Column B. You may use an answer more than once.

COLUMN A

_____ 1. ferrous sulfate

_____ 2. epoetin alfa

_____ 3. folic acid

_____ 4. iron sucrose

_____ 5. sodium ferric gluconate

_____ 6. vitamin B_{12}

_____ 7. darbepoetin alfa

_____ 8. ferrous fumarate

COLUMN B

A. Anemia associated with chronic renal failure.
B. Iron deficiency anemia.
C. Megaloblastic anemia.
D. B_{12} deficiency.

III. MATCHING

Match the type of anticoagulant in Column A with the drug name in Column B. You may use an answer more than once.

COLUMN A

_____ 1. enoxaparin sodium

_____ 2. heparin

_____ 3. protamine sulfate

_____ 4. anisindione

_____ 5. warfarin sodium

_____ 6. danaparoid sodium

_____ 7. dalteparin sodium

_____ 8. tinzaparin sodium

_____ 9. phytonadione

COLUMN B

A. Coumadin
B. indandione derivative
C. unfractionated heparin
D. fractionated heparin
E. anticoagulant antagonist

IV. MATCHING

Match the generic anticoagulant or thrombolytic in Column A with the trade name in Column B.

COLUMN A

_____ 1. anisindione

_____ 2. dalteparin sodium

_____ 3. urokinase

_____ 4. danaparoid sodium

_____ 5. alteplase

_____ 6. enoxaparin sodium

_____ 7. tinzaparin sodium

_____ 8. streptokinase

_____ 9. warfarin sodium

_____ 10. phytonadione

COLUMN B

A. Coumadin
B. Lovenox
C. Innohep
D. Fragmin
E. Aqua-MEPHYTON
F. Orgaran
G. Activase
H. Abbokinase
I. Miradon
J. Streptase

V. TRUE/FALSE

Indicate whether each statement is True (T) or False (F).

_____ 1. Anticoagulant therapy can prevent clots from forming.

_____ 2. Thrombolytic drugs can prevent the formation of a thrombus.

_____ 3. The most common adverse reaction of warfarin sodium is bleeding.

_____ 4. Warfarin sodium overdoses may be treated by administering vitamin K.

_____ 5. Warfarin sodium may safely be used during pregnancy and lactation.

_____ 6. Heparin is not a single drug.

_____ 7. Clotting is the chief complication of heparin administration.

_____ 8. LMWHs cause fewer adverse reactions than heparin.

_____ 9. Protamine sulfate counteracts the effects of heparin.

_____ 10. Heparin must be given by the parenteral route.

_____ 11. LMWHs are only given in the hospital, but heparin can be administered at home.

_____ 12. Thrombolytics dissolve certain types of blood clots and can reopen vessels after they have been occluded.

_____ 13. The most common adverse reaction caused by thrombolytic drug use is bleeding.

_____ 14. Iron preparations act by depleting iron stores.

_____ 15. An adverse reaction of oral iron preparations is constipation.

_____ 16. Hypersensitivity reactions have never been reported with the use of parenteral iron.

_____ 17. Patients with uncontrolled hypertension should not be prescribed either epoetin alfa or darbepoetin alfa.

_____ 18. Leucovorin calcium increases the effectiveness of anticonvulsants.

_____ 19. Vitamin B_{12} therapy is contraindicated in patients allergic to cobalt.

VI. MULTIPLE CHOICE

Circle the letter of the best answer.

1. Anticoagulants _____ .
   a. have no direct effect on an existing thrombus
   b. do not reverse any damage from a thrombus
   c. can prevent additional clots from forming
   d. are sometimes called blood thinners
   e. all of the answers are correct

2. All of the following drugs are anticoagulants except _____ .
   a. warfarin sodium
   b. streptokinase
   c. anisindione
   d. fractionated heparin (LMWH)
   e. unfractionated heparin (heparin sodium)

3. Warfarin sodium _____ .
   a. interferes with the production of vitamin K-dependent clotting factors
   b. works better if given with vitamin C
   c. prevents the formation of erythropoietin by the kidneys
   d. is contraindicated in patients with iron deficiency anemia
   e. can produce a decrease in the effectiveness of leucovorin calcium

4. Mr. S is currently taking warfarin sodium. His last PT and INR were within therapeutic range. He called into his healthcare provider's office this afternoon saying that his gums are still bleeding after brushing his teeth this morning. As the healthcare worker who took the call you should _____ .

a. tell him to buy a soft toothbrush
b. tell him not to worry, this is normal
c. tell him not to brush his teeth
d. report this immediately to the healthcare provider
e. tell him to call back in a few days if he continues to bleed

5. Diet can influence the effectiveness of warfarin sodium therapy. It is best for patients taking warfarin sodium to _____ .

a. eat a diet high in vitamin K
b. eat a diet low in vitamin K
c. eat a diet with a consistent amount of vitamin K
d. totally eliminate vitamin K from their diet
e. change to injection-administered warfarin sodium

6. All of the following are true regarding heparin except _____ .

a. may be given orally
b. inhibits the formation of fibrin clots
c. inhibits the conversion of fibrinogen to fibrin
d. has no effects on existing cells
e. inactivates several factors needed for clotting

7. Heparin administration can cause bleeding which _____ .

a. can be at any site
b. is more common in individuals older than 60
c. is more common in women
d. should be reported immediately to the healthcare provider
e. all of the answers are correct

8. LMWHs are contraindicated in all of the following patients except _____ .

a. those with a known hypersensitivity to the drug or heparin
b. those with deep vein thrombosis
c. those with a known hypersensitivity to pork products
d. those with thrombocytopenia
e. those with active bleeding

9. All of the following will increase the effects of heparin when administered together except _____ .

a. NSAIDs
b. aspirin
c. penicillin
d. protamine sulfate
e. cephalosporin

10. Thrombolytic drugs work by _____ .

a. breaking down prothrombin
b. converting plasminogen to plasmin
c. forming fibrin clots
d. converting prothrombin to thrombin
e. none of the answers are correct

11. Patients being treated with thrombolytic drugs _____ .

a. should not be given an anticoagulant
b. cannot have had recent intracranial surgery
c. should be physically active
d. should be monitored for signs of bleeding and hemorrhage
e. answers b and d are correct

12. Thrombolytic drugs work best to dissolve thrombi when they are _____ .

a. given as soon as possible after the formation of a thrombus
b. given within 4 to 6 hours after the formation of a thrombus
c. given within 24 hours after the formation of a thrombus
d. given in conjunction with protamine sulfate
e. injected directly into the thrombus

13. Which parenteral iron preparation is used for the treatment of iron deficiency anemia when oral treatments cannot be used because of gastrointestinal intolerance?

a. ferrous sulfate
b. iron dextran
c. ferrous gluconate
d. ferrous fumarate
e. iron sucrose

14. Iron compounds are contraindicated in which of the following patients?

a. patients with any anemia except iron deficiency anemia
b. patients with a known hypersensitivity to the drug
c. patients with sulfate sensitivity
d. patients with cardiovascular disease
e. answers a and b are correct

15. Epoetin alfa is used to treat _____ .

a. anemia caused by chemotherapy
b. anemia of chronic renal failure
c. anemia in patients undergoing elective nonvascular surgery
d. answers a and c are correct
e. answers a, b, and c are correct

16. Darbepoetin _____ .
   a. acts by stimulating erythropoiesis
   b. elevates or maintains RBC levels
   c. decreases the need for transfusions
   d. can be used to treat anemia caused by chronic renal failure
   e. all of the answers are correct

17. All of the following are correct regarding leucovorin calcium except that it _____ .
   a. uses a derivative of folic acid
   b. can be administered orally or parenterally
   c. can be used to rescue normal cells from methotrexate
   d. it can be used safely in patients with pernicious anemia
   e. has few adverse reactions

VII. RECALL FACTS

Indicate which of the following statements are Facts with an F. If the statement is not a fact, leave the line blank.

About Medications That May Cause an Increase in the Effect of Warfarin Sodium

_____ 1. oral contraceptives

_____ 2. acetaminophen

_____ 3. ascorbic acid

_____ 4. barbiturates

_____ 5. beta blockers

_____ 6. diuretics

_____ 7. aminoglycosides

_____ 8. tetracyclines

_____ 9. vitamin K

_____ 10. NSAIDs

_____ 11. cephalosporins

_____ 12. loop diuretics

About Situations in Which Heparin Is Used

_____ 1. Atrial fibrillation with embolus formation

_____ 2. Prevention of clotting in medical equipment

_____ 3. Treatment of DIC

_____ 4. Labor and delivery

_____ 5. Prevention of clotting in arterial and heart surgery

_____ 6. Destruction of clots already formed

VIII. FILL IN THE BLANK

Fill in the blanks using words from the list below.

clot formation	drop
PT	INR
1.5	rise
drop	APTT
10	4
1	increases
depletes	decrease
elevating	3
bleeding	6

1. The healthcare provider should be notified immediately if a patient taking warfarin sodium has a(n) _____ greater than _____ times the control value, has a(n) _____ greater than _____, or has evidence of _____ .

2. Vitamin K administration will enhance _____ and return the PT to an acceptable level in approximately _____ hours.

3. A significant _____ in blood pressure or a _____ in pulse rate may indicate internal bleeding.

4. The laboratory test used to manage warfarin sodium therapy is the _____, whereas the _____ test is used to monitor heparin therapy.

5. Heparin causes anticoagulation after _____ dose, with maximum effects within _____ minutes, but the clotting time will return to normal within _____ hours unless additional doses are given.

6. Iron preparations act by _____ the serum iron concentration, which replenishes hemoglobin and _____ iron stores.

7. Ascorbic acid _____ the absorption of oral iron, whereas antacids _____ oral iron absorption.

IX. LIST

List the requested number of items.

1. List five uses of warfarin sodium.

   a. _____
   b. _____
   c. _____
   d. _____
   e. _____

2. List four symptoms of overdosage of warfarin sodium.

   a. _____
   b. _____
   c. _____
   d. _____

3. List six common cooking herbs warfarin sodium should not be combined with because of the additive effects and increased risk of bleeding.

   a. _____
   b. _____
   c. _____
   d. _____
   e. _____
   f. _____

4. List six conditions in which heparin therapy is contraindicated.

   a. _____
   b. _____
   c. _____
   d. _____
   e. _____
   f. _____

5. List four uses of thrombolytic drugs.

   a. _____
   b. _____
   c. _____
   d. _____

6. List four adverse reactions that when present while administering parenteral iron need to be reported to the healthcare provider.

   a. _____
   b. _____
   c. _____
   d. _____

7. List four types of patients in whom a vitamin B_{12} deficiency may be seen.

   a. _____
   b. _____
   c. _____
   d. _____

X. CLINICAL APPLICATIONS

1. Mr. F has chronic renal failure and is undergoing dialysis twice weekly for this condition. Anemia has developed as a result of his kidneys failing to produce adequate amounts of erythropoietin. Choose the best drug to treat Mr. F's anemia and explain the drug's action.

2. Mrs. G was hospitalized with deep vein thrombosis 2 weeks ago and was sent home with a prescription for warfarin sodium. Her current INR is 2.7. What information should Mrs. G be aware of while taking warfarin sodium?

19 Diuretics

I. MATCHING

Match the term from Column A with the correct definition from Column B.

COLUMN A

_____ 1. diuretic

_____ 2. edema

_____ 3. hyperkalemia

_____ 4. hypokalemia

_____ 5. orthostatic hypotension

_____ 6. postural hypotension

COLUMN B

A. Dizziness or light-headedness when rising suddenly from a sitting or lying position.
B. High blood level of potassium.
C. Retention of excess fluid.
D. Dizziness and light-headedness after standing in one place for a long time.
E. Low blood level of potassium.
F. A drug that increases the secretion of urine by the kidneys.

II. MATCHING

Match the generic diuretic from Column A with the correct trade name from Column B.

COLUMN A

_____ 1. torsemide

_____ 2. bumetanide

_____ 3. glycerin

_____ 4. triamterene

_____ 5. mannitol

_____ 6. amiloride

_____ 7. furosemide

_____ 8. indapamide

_____ 9. chlorothiazide

_____ 10. polythiazide

COLUMN B

A. Osmitrol
B. Osmoglyn
C. Lasix
D. Lozol
E. Demadex
F. Diuril
G. Midamor
H. Renese
I. Bumex
J. Dyrenium

III. MATCHING

Match the trade name from Column A with the correct type of diuretic from Column B. You may use an answer more than once.

COLUMN A

_____ 1. Hygroton

_____ 2. Aldactone

_____ 3. Edecrin

_____ 4. Exna

_____ 5. Diamox

_____ 6. Demadex

_____ 7. Naturetin

_____ 8. Diurese

_____ 9. Hydromox

_____ 10. Dyrenium

_____ 11. Neptazane

_____ 12. Ismotic

COLUMN B

A. Carbonic anhydrase inhibitor
B. Loop diuretic
C. Osmotic diuretic
D. Potassium-sparing diuretic
E. Thiazides and related diuretics

IV. TRUE/FALSE

Indicate whether each statement is True (T) or False (F).

_____ 1. Diuretics are only used to treat hypertension.

_____ 2. Carbonic anhydrase inhibitors can be used to treat glaucoma.

_____ 3. Adverse reactions associated with short-term therapy with carbonic anhydrase inhibitors are rare.

_____ 4. Loop diuretics work by increasing the excretion of sodium and chloride by stimulating their reabsorption in the proximal and distal tubules and in the loop of Henle.

_____ 5. Torsemide acts primarily in the ascending portion of the loop of Henle.

_____ 6. Bumex acts primarily on the proximal tubule of the nephron.

_____ 7. Patients with diabetes who take loop diuretics may experience a decrease in blood glucose levels.

_____ 8. A potential adverse reaction of loop diuretics is orthostatic hypertension.

_____ 9. It is safe to give infants ethacrynic acid.

_____ 10. A patient who is sensitive to the sulfonamides may have an allergic reaction to Bumex.

_____ 11. Osmotic diuretics increase the density of the filtrate in the glomerulus.

_____ 12. Osmotic diuretics only allow water to be excreted.

_____ 13. Aldactone antagonizes the action of aldosterone.

_____ 14. Potassium-sparing diuretics may cause hyperkalemia in patients with inadequate fluid intake.

_____ 15. All potassium-sparing diuretics are Pregnancy Category B drugs.

_____ 16. Cardiac arrest may occur when a patient taking a potassium preparation is administered a potassium-sparing diuretic.

_____ 17. Thiazides work by inhibiting the reabsorption of sodium and chloride ions.

_____ 18. The electrolyte and fluid loss associated with thiazide use can often be easily corrected.

_____ 19. All thiazide diuretics are Pregnancy Category B drugs.

_____ 20. The duration of activity of most diuretics is 8 hours or less.

_____ 21. The most common electrolyte imbalances experienced by patients taking a diuretic are the loss of potassium and water.

_____ 22. Older adults should be monitored for hypokalemia when taking a potassium-sparing diuretic.

_____ 23. Most herbal diuretics are either ineffective or no more effective than caffeine.

V. MULTIPLE CHOICE

Circle the letter of the best answer.

1. Carbonic anhydrase inhibitors work by _____ .
   a. inhibiting the action of the enzyme carbonic anhydrase
   b. increasing the production of the enzyme carbonic anhydrase
   c. decreasing the production of the enzyme carbonic anhydrase
   d. stimulating the action of the enzyme carbonic anhydrase
   e. none of the answers are correct

2. Carbonic anhydrase inhibitors have the effect of excretion of _____ by the kidneys.
   a. sodium
   b. potassium
   c. bicarbonate
   d. water
   e. all of the answers are correct

3. _____, a carbonic anhydrase inhibitor, is used in the treatment of simple (open-angle) glaucoma and secondary glaucoma.
   a. Neptazane
   b. Diamox
   c. Bumex
   d. Ismotic
   e. Edecrin

4. All of the following, except one, are patients in whom carbonic anhydrase inhibitors would be contraindicated. Which is the exception?

   a. patients with electrolyte imbalances
   b. patients with severe kidney dysfunction
   c. patients with asthma
   d. patients with anuria
   e. patients with liver dysfunction

5. _____ is an example of a loop diuretic.

   a. Furosemide
   b. Acetazolamide
   c. Ethacrynic acid
   d. Answers a and c are correct
   e. All of the answers are correct

6. _____ can be used for the short-term management of ascites.

   a. Furosemide
   b. Torsemide
   c. Bumetanide
   d. Ethacrynic acid
   e. Mannitol

7. Which loop diuretic is a Pregnancy Category C drug?

   a. ethacrynic acid
   b. furosemide
   c. torsemide
   d. answers b and c are correct
   e. all of the answers are correct

8. Ototoxicity can occur if a loop diuretic is given with a _____ .

   a. thrombolytic
   b. aminoglycoside
   c. cardiac drug
   d. NSAID
   e. lithium drug

9. Loop diuretics may increase the effectiveness of which of the following drugs?

   a. thrombolytics
   b. anticoagulants
   c. propranolol
   d. lithium
   e. all of the answers are correct

10. _____ is an osmotic diuretic that is administered intravenously.

   a. Urea
   b. Glycerin
   c. Mannitol
   d. Isosorbide
   e. Answers a and c are correct

11. Which of the following osmotic diuretics is a Pregnancy Category B drug?

   a. glycerin
   b. mannitol
   c. isosorbide
   d. urea
   e. answers b and d are correct

12. Triamterene is a(n) _____ .

   a. osmotic diuretic
   b. potassium-sparing diuretic
   c. loop diuretic
   d. thiazide
   e. carbonic anhydrase inhibitor

13. Potassium-sparing diuretics are used to treat _____ .

   a. chronic heart failure
   b. hypertension
   c. edema caused by chronic heart failure
   d. answers a and c are correct
   e. all of the answers are correct

14. In which of the following patients are potassium-sparing diuretics contraindicated?

   a. patients with hyperkalemia
   b. patients with anuria
   c. patients with significant renal impairment
   d. patients with serious electrolyte imbalances
   e. all of the answers are correct

15. Administration of a thiazide will result in the _____ .

   a. retention of potassium
   b. excretion of potassium
   c. excretion of sodium, chloride, and water
   d. retention of sodium, chloride, and water
   e. none of the answers are correct

16. Some thiazides contain _____, which may cause bronchial asthma in patients who are sensitive to the drug.

   a. tartrazine
   b. theophylline
   c. aminoglycosides
   d. penicillin
   e. glucose

17. Patients taking thiazides or related diuretics may experience _____ as an adverse reaction.

   a. azotemia
   b. gout
   c. hyperglycemia
   d. all of the answers are correct
   e. none of the answers are correct

VI. RECALL FACTS

Indicate which of the following statements are Facts with an F. If the statement is not a fact, leave the line blank.

About Those Instances in Which Concurrent Thiazide Administration Will Increase the Other Drug's Effects

_____ 1. Allopurinol hypersensitivity

_____ 2. Anticoagulant effects

_____ 3. Antidiabetic drugs

_____ 4. Anesthetics

_____ 5. Uric acid levels

_____ 6. Glycoside toxicity

VII. FILL IN THE BLANK

Fill in the blanks using words from the list below.

renal dysfunction   mannitol
electrolyte imbalance   tubules
chloride   gynecomastia
2 pounds   cardiac arrhythmias
avoided   C
furosemide   increased
reabsorption   excretion
hypokalemia   hourly
sulfonamides

1. Most diuretics act on the _____ of the kidney nephron.

2. Diuretics are Pregnancy Category _____ drugs.

3. Patients taking carbonic anhydrase inhibitors have a(n) _____ risk of cyclosporine toxicity when the drug is administered with acetazolamide.

4. Bumex primarily increases the excretion of _____ .

5. _____ is the drug of choice when rapid diuresis is needed.

6. Loop diuretics are used cautiously in patients with _____ .

7. When administered to a patient in a fasting state, osmotic diuretics may result in a rapid _____ .

8. _____ is contraindicated in patients with active intracranial bleeding.

9. Midamor acts by depressing the _____ of sodium and by depressing the _____ of potassium.

10. _____ may occur in patients taking spironolactone.

11. A cross-sensitivity reaction may occur with thiazides and _____ .

12. Mannitol requires _____ monitoring of urine output.

13. In patients with edema who are being treated with a diuretic, a weight loss of approximately _____ per day is desirable.

14. An older adult is monitored for _____ if taking a loop or thiazide diuretic.

15. Patients concurrently receiving a diuretic and a digitalis glycoside require frequent monitoring for _____ .

16. Diuretic teas should be _____ .

VIII. LIST

List the requested number of items.

1. List five types of diuretic drugs.

   a. _____

   b. _____

   c. _____

   d. _____

   e. _____

2. List five adverse reactions caused by long-term use of carbonic anhydrase inhibitors.

a. _____

b. _____

c. _____

d. _____

e. _____

3. List three uses of loop diuretics.

a. _____

b. _____

c. _____

4. List three uses of osmotic diuretics.

a. _____

b. _____

c. _____

5. List four trade names of osmotic diuretic drugs.

a. _____

b. _____

c. _____

d. _____

6. List five types of patients in whom hyperkalemia may occur when treated with a potassium-sparing diuretic.

a. _____

b. _____

c. _____

d. _____

e. _____

7. List two uses of thiazides.

a. _____

b. _____

8. List five symptoms of hyperkalemia.

a. _____

b. _____

c. _____

d. _____

e. _____

9. List five warning signs of fluid and electrolyte imbalance.

a. _____

b. _____

c. _____

d. _____

e. _____

10. List five herbal diuretics.

a. _____

b. _____

c. _____

d. _____

e. _____

IX. CLINICAL APPLICATION

1. Mrs. K, age 63, has been diagnosed with chronic heart failure. As a result of this condition, she has edema, which must be treated immediately. Using your text as a guide, answer the following questions.

a. Which type of diuretic would most likely be chosen to treat Mrs. K's edema?

b. Which specific drug is the drug of choice when rapid diuresis is required?

c. What is the most common adverse reaction associated with diuretics?

20 Urinary Anti-Infectives and Miscellaneous Urinary Drugs

I. MATCHING

Match the term from Column A with the correct definition from Column B.

COLUMN A

_____ 1. dysuria

_____ 2. neurogenic bladder

_____ 3. overactive bladder

_____ 4. urge incontinence

_____ 5. urinary frequency

_____ 6. urinary urgency

COLUMN B

A. Painful or difficult urination.
B. Frequent urination day and night.
C. Strong sudden need to urinate.
D. Involuntary contractions of the detrusor or bladder muscle.
E. Altered bladder function caused by a nervous system abnormality.
F. Accidental loss of urine caused by a sudden and unstoppable need to urinate.

II. MATCHING

Match the generic drug name from Column A with the correct trade name from Column B.

COLUMN A

_____ 1. nalidixic acid

_____ 2. nitrofurantoin macrocrystals

_____ 3. sulfamethizole

_____ 4. phenazopyridine

_____ 5. oxybutynin chloride

_____ 6. cinoxacin

_____ 7. methenamine hippurate

_____ 8. tolterodine tartrate

_____ 9. nitrofurantoin

_____ 10. flavoxate HCl

_____ 11. trimethoprim (TMP)

_____ 12. trimethoprim and sulfamethoxazole (TMP-SMZ)

COLUMN B

A. Urispas
B. NegGram
C. Detrol
D. Bactrim
E. Hiprex
F. Thiosulfil Forte
G. Furadantin
H. Ditropan
I. Cinobac
J. Proloprim
K. Macrobid
L. Pyridate

III. MATCHING

Match the drug trade name from Column A with the type of drug from Column B. You may use an answer more than once.

COLUMN A

_____ 1. Urogesic

_____ 2. Thiosulfil Forte

_____ 3. Macrobid

_____ 4. NegGram

_____ 5. Urispas

_____ 6. Mandelamine

_____ 7. Detrol

_____ 8. Bactrim

_____ 9. Monurol

_____ 10. Ditropan

COLUMN B

A. Anti-infective drug
B. Miscellaneous urinary drug
C. Urinary anti-infective combination drug

IV. TRUE/FALSE

Indicate whether each statement is True (T) or False (F).

_____ 1. Urinary anti-infectives that are taken by the oral or parenteral route do not achieve significant levels in the bloodstream.

_____ 2. Cinoxacin is effective against susceptible Gram-negative bacteria.

_____ 3. Ammonia and formaldehyde formed from the breakdown of methenamine and methenamine salts are bactericidal.

_____ 4. Visual disturbances that can occur after nalidixic acid administration can become permanent.

_____ 5. Nitrofurantoin may be bacteriostatic or bactericidal.

_____ 6. Fosfomycin is bactericidal.

_____ 7. Flavoxate causes contraction of the detrusor muscle through action at the sympathetic receptors of the bladder.

_____ 8. Flavoxate can cause mental confusion in elderly patients.

_____ 9. Pyridium is a dye that has no anti-infective activity.

_____ 10. Detrol is used to treat symptoms of overactive bladder.

_____ 11. Pulmonary reactions have been reported with the use of nitrofurantoin.

_____ 12. Phenazopyridine causes permanent reddish-orange discoloration of the urine.

_____ 13. No serious drug interactions have been reported with methenamine.

V. MULTIPLE CHOICE

Circle the letter of the best answer.

1. Which of the following is not considered to be an adverse reaction of cinoxacin?
   a. nausea
   b. rash
   c. abdominal pain
   d. photophobia
   e. perineal burning

2. Large doses of methenamine may result in _____ .
   a. cystitis
   b. bladder irritation
   c. burning on urination
   d. answers a and b are correct
   e. answers b and c are correct

3. Nalidixic acid appears to act by _____ .
   a. interrupting bacterial RNA replication
   b. lysing the bacterial cell wall
   c. interfering with bacterial multiplication
   d. inhibiting the metabolism of glucose
   e. none of the answers are correct

4. Fosfomycin acts by _____ .
   a. lysing the bacterial cell wall
   b. interfering with the metabolism of dextrose
   c. interrupting RNA replication
   d. interfering with cell wall synthesis
   e. answers a and c are correct

5. Nausea can be an adverse reaction to _____ .
   a. nitrofurantoin
   b. fosfomycin
   c. trimethoprim
   d. flavoxate
   e. all of the answers are correct

6. _____ is used to treat bladder instability caused by a neurogenic bladder.
   a. Pyridium
   b. Ditropan
   c. Detrol
   d. Urispas
   e. Trimpex

7. _____ is an anticholinergic drug that inhibits bladder contractions.
   a. Tolterodine
   b. Phenazopyridine
   c. Oxybutynin
   d. Flavoxate
   e. Nitrofurantoin

8. Nitrofurantoin may cause a(n) _____ which needs to be reported to the healthcare provider and the next dose is not taken until the patient is evaluated.
   a. blood glucose elevation
   b. severe arrhythmia
   c. permanent visual disturbance
   d. pulmonary reaction
   e. ototoxicity reaction

9. _____ is contraindicated in patients with gastric blockage, abdominal bleeding, or urinary tract blockage.

    a. Oxybutynin
    b. Flavoxate
    c. Phenazopyridine
    d. Nitrofurantoin
    e. Trimethoprim

10. When haloperidol is administered with _____, there is an increased risk of tardive dyskinesia.

    a. Oxybutynin
    b. Flavoxate
    c. Phenazopyridine
    d. Nitrofurantoin
    e. Trimethoprim

11. Cranberries _____ .

    a. inhibit bacteria from attaching to the walls of the urinary tract
    b. prevent certain bacteria from forming dental plaque in the mouth
    c. have no known adverse reactions
    d. have no known drug interactions
    e. all of the answers are correct

VI. FILL IN THE BLANK

Fill in the blanks using words from the list below.

analgesic	Trimpex
methenamine	urine
dry mouth	antacids
megaloblastic anemia	cinoxacin
urine	

1. Urinary anti-infective drugs exert their major antibacterial effects in the _____ .

2. _____ acts by disrupting the replication of DNA in susceptible bacteria.

3. _____ breaks down to form ammonia and formaldehyde.

4. Nitrofurantoin's mode of action is dependent on the concentration of the drug in the _____ .

5. _____ acts by interfering with the metabolism of folinic acid by the bacteria.

6. Phenazopyridine is a urinary _____ drug.

7. The most common adverse reaction of tolterodine is _____ .

8. When taking methenamine the patient should not use _____ containing sodium bicarbonate or sodium carbonate.

9. Trimethoprim is used with caution in patients with _____ caused by folate deficiency.

VII. LIST

List the requested number of items.

1. List five trade names of urinary anti-infective drugs.

    a. _____
    b. _____
    c. _____
    d. _____
    e. _____

2. List six conditions that Urispas is used to treat.

    a. _____
    b. _____
    c. _____
    d. _____
    e. _____
    f. _____

3. List four conditions in which nalidixic acid should be used with caution.

    a. _____
    b. _____
    c. _____
    d. _____

VIII. CLINICAL APPLICATION

1. Miss P was told that drinking a glass of cranberry juice everyday will cure her urinary tract infection. Explain to Miss P the role that cranberry juice can play in the treatment of her infection.

21 Drugs That Affect the Gastrointestinal System

I. MATCHING

Match the term from Column A with the correct definition from Column B.

COLUMN A

_____ 1. emetic

_____ 2. gallstone-solubilizing

_____ 3. gastric stasis

_____ 4. hypersecretory

_____ 5. paralytic ileus

_____ 6. proton pump inhibitors

COLUMN B

A. Gallstone dissolving
B. Failure to move food normally out of the stomach
C. Excessive gastric secretion of hydrochloric acid
D. A drug that induces vomiting
E. Drugs with antisecretory properties

II. MATCHING

Match the generic proton pump inhibitor or miscellaneous gastrointestinal drug from Column A with the correct trade name from Column B.

COLUMN A

_____ 1. sucralfate

_____ 2. mesalamine

_____ 3. sulfasalazine

_____ 4. omeprazole

_____ 5. rabeprazole sodium

_____ 6. esomeprazole magnesium

_____ 7. misoprostol

_____ 8. infliximab

_____ 9. olsalazine

_____ 10. lansoprazole

COLUMN B

A. Azulfidine
B. Aciphex
C. Prevacid
D. Carafate
E. Cytotec
F. Dipentum
G. Remicade
H. Asacol
I. Nexium
J. Prilosec

III. MATCHING

Match the generic antacid or anticholinergic drug name from Column A with the correct trade name from Column B.

COLUMN A

_____ 1. calcium carbonate

_____ 2. mepenzolate bromide

_____ 3. glycopyrrolate

_____ 4. aluminum carbonate gel

_____ 5. tridihexethyl chloride

_____ 6. clindinium bromide

_____ 7. aluminum hydroxide gel

_____ 8. dicyclomine HCl

_____ 9. magnesia

_____ 10. propantheline bromide

_____ 11. magaldrate

_____ 12. methantheline bromide

COLUMN B

A. Chooz
B. Quarzan
C. Banthine
D. Bentyl
E. Riopan
F. Cantil
G. Basaljel
H. Robinul

I. Alu-Tab
J. Pathilon
K. Milk of Magnesia
L. Pro-Banthine

IV. MATCHING

Match the generic gastrointestinal stimulant, hista-mine H_2 antagonist, antidiarrheal, or antiflatulent drug from Column A with the correct trade name in Column B.

COLUMN A

_____ 1. dexpanthenol

_____ 2. famotidine

_____ 3. simethicone

_____ 4. metoclopramide

_____ 5. ranitidine

_____ 6. diphenoxylate HCl

_____ 7. nizatidine

_____ 8. L-hyoscyamine sulfate

_____ 9. cimetidine

_____ 10. loperamide HCl

COLUMN B

A. Zantac
B. Imodium A-D
C. Tagamet
D. Lomotil
E. Pepcid
F. Reglan
G. Axid Pulvules
H. Anaspaz
I. Gas-X
J. Ilopan

V. MATCHING

Match the generic digestive enzyme, emetic, gallstone-solubilizing agent, or bowel evacuant drug name from Column A with the correct trade name from Column B.

COLUMN A

_____ 1. pancreatin

_____ 2. polyethylene glycol

_____ 3. amorphine HCl

_____ 4. ursodiol

_____ 5. pancrelipase

_____ 6. polyethylene glycol electrolyte solution

COLUMN B

A. Actigall
B. MiraLax
C. CoLyte
D. Cotazym Capsules
E. amorphine HCl
F. Creon

VI. MATCHING

Match the generic laxative name from Column A with the correct trade name from Column B.

COLUMN A

_____ 1. glycerin

_____ 2. docusate calcium

_____ 3. psyllium

_____ 4. docusate sodium

_____ 5. sennosides

_____ 6. magnesium preparations

_____ 7. lactulose

_____ 8. polycarbophil

COLUMN B

A. Colace
B. Metamucil
C. Chronulac
D. Epsom Salt
E. Senokot
F. Colace Suppositories
G. FiberCon
H. Surfak Liquigels

VII. MATCHING

Match he trade name from Column A with the correct type of drug from Column B. You may use an answer more than once.

COLUMN A

_____ 1. Reglan

_____ 2. Remicade

_____ 3. Pamine

_____ 4. Imodium A-D

_____ 5. Prevacid

_____ 6. ipecac syrup

_____ 7. Riopan

_____ 8. Tagamet

_____ 9. Actigall

_____ 10. Dipentum

_____ 11. MiraLax

_____ 12. Quarzan

_____ 13. Metamucil

_____ 14. Pepcid

_____ 15. Colace

_____ 16. Prilosec

_____ 17. Digepepsin

_____ 18. Ex-Lax

_____ 19. Tums

_____ 20. Mylicon

COLUMN B

A. Proton pump inhibitor
B. Miscellaneous gastrointestinal drug
C. Antacid
D. Anticholinergic
E. Gastrointestinal stimulant
F. Histamine H_2 antagonist
G. Antidiarrheal
H. Antiflatulent
I. Digestive enzyme
J. Emetic
K. Gallstone-solubilizing agent
L. Laxative
M. Bowel evacuant

VIII. MATCHING

Match the miscellaneous gastrointestinal drug from Column A with the correct drug action from Column B. You may use an answer more than once.

COLUMN A

_____ 1. misoprostol

_____ 2. sucralfate

_____ 3. mesalamine

_____ 4. olsalazine

_____ 5. sulfasalazine

_____ 6. bismuth subsalicylate

COLUMN B

A. Topical anti-inflammatory effect
B. Local action on lining of the stomach
C. Inhibits gastric acid secretion and increases mucus production
D. Disrupts the integrity of bacterial cell walls

IX. TRUE/FALSE

Indicate whether each statement is True (T) or False (F).

_____ 1. Antacids work by changing the hydrochloric acid in the stomach to a base.

_____ 2. Antacids can be used to treat other conditions not related to an acidic stomach.

_____ 3. Oral iron products have a decreased pharmacological effect when administered with an antacid.

_____ 4. Anticholinergics reduce gastric motility.

_____ 5. Histamine H_2 antagonists have more adverse reactions than anticholinergic drugs when used to treat peptic ulcers.

_____ 6. Reglan and Ilopan decrease the strength of spontaneous movement of the upper gastrointestinal tract and are used in the treatment of diarrhea.

_____ 7. Dexpanthenol administration may cause itching, difficulty breathing, and urticaria.

_____ 8. Gastrointestinal stimulants are secreted in breast milk.

_____ 9. Tardive dyskinesia as a result of gastrointestinal stimulant therapy is reversible.

_____ 10. When Tagamet is given concurrently with morphine, the patient has an increased risk of respiratory depression.

_____ 11. Motofen increases intestinal peristalsis.

_____ 12. Antidiarrheals are contraindicated in children who are younger than 2 years of age.

_____ 13. Charcoal works as an antiflatulent by reducing the amount of intestinal gas.

_____ 14. Many adverse reactions have been reported by patients who have received an antiflatulent.

_____ 15. Simethicone has no known drug interactions.

_____ 16. Digestive enzymes are prescribed for patients with an overactive pancreas.

_____ 17. Patients with acute pancreatitis should be prescribed high doses of digestive enzymes.

_____ 18. Radiolucent gallstones may decrease in size when a patient is given Actigall.

_____ 19. Hepatotoxicity may be an adverse reaction of prolonged use of gallstone-solubilizing drugs.

_____ 20. Calcified gallstones can be safely treated with ursodiol.

_____ 21. The action of all laxatives is the same.

_____ 22. Mineral oil, when used as a laxative, can cause impairment of fat-soluble vitamin absorption.

_____ 23. Proton pump inhibitors work by suppressing gastric acid secretion.

_____ 24. Bismuth subsalicylate can cause salicylate toxicity if used for an extended period.

_____ 25. Chamomile is safe for all patients to take when the oral form is used.

X. MULTIPLE CHOICE

Circle the letter of the best answer.

1. In which of the following conditions are antacids used as part of the treatment regimen?
   a. acid indigestion
   b. sour stomach
   c. peptic ulcer
   d. heartburn
   e. all of the answers are correct

2. An antacid that contains magnesium may produce _____ as an adverse reaction.
   a. constipation
   b. anorexia
   c. dehydration
   d. metabolic alkalosis
   e. renal calculi

3. A calcium-containing antacid may produce _____ as an adverse reaction.
   a. rebound hypersecretion
   b. neurologic impairment
   c. severe diarrhea
   d. bone pain
   e. tremors

4. Which type of patient should not take a sodium-containing antacid?
   a. a patient with renal calculi
   b. a patient with a gastric outlet obstruction
   c. a patient with respiratory insufficiency
   d. a patient with congestive heart failure
   e. a patient with decreased kidney function

5. Which of the following drugs would have a decreased pharmacological effect when administered with an antacid?
   a. tetracycline
   b. valproic acid
   c. phenytoin
   d. ranitidine
   e. all of the answers are correct

6. Which gastrointestinal stimulant may be given IV immediately after major abdominal surgery to reduce the risk of paralytic ileus?
   a. dexpanthenol
   b. metoclopramide
   c. famotidine
   d. ranitidine
   e. cimetidine

7. Patients receiving high or prolonged doses of metoclopramide should be monitored for symptoms of _____ .
   a. extrapyramidal reactions
   b. tardive dyskinesia
   c. shortness of breath
   d. answers a and b are correct
   e. all of the answers are correct

8. Histamine H_2 antagonists _____ .
   a. inhibit the action of histamine in the stomach
   b. decrease total pepsin output
   c. reduce the secretions of gastric acid
   d. answers a and c are correct
   e. all of the answers are correct

9. Which of the following is not an example of a histamine H_2 antagonist?
   a. Reglan
   b. Zantac

c. Tagamet
d. Pepcid
e. Axid Pulvules

10. In which of the following patients are histamine H_2 antagonists contraindicated?

a. a patient with diabetes
b. a patient with renal impairment
c. a patient with a known hypersensitivity
d. a patient with hepatic impairment
e. all of the answers are correct

11. With which of the following drugs, when given concurrently with a histamine H_2 antagonist, does the patient have an increased risk of toxicity?

a. oral anticoagulant
b. phenytoin
c. quinidine
d. lidocaine
e. all of the answers are correct

12. Loperamide is an example of a(n) _____ .

a. gastrointestinal stimulant
b. antidiarrheal
c. histamine H_2 antagonist
d. antacid
e. antiflatulent

13. _____ is a narcotic-related drug that is used for the treatment of diarrhea and has a potential for drug dependency.

a. Difenoxin
b. Diphenoxylate
c. Atropine
d. Loperamide
e. Simethicone

14. Antidiarrheals are contraindicated in which of the following patients?

a. patients with pseudomembranous colitis
b. patients with abdominal pain of unknown origin
c. patients with obstructive jaundice
d. patients with *Escherichia coli*, *Salmonella*, or *Shigella* infections
e. all of the answers are correct

15. Charcoal may be used as a(n) _____ .

a. antiflatulent
b. antidote in poisoning
c. method of preventing nonspecific pruritus
d. answers a and b are correct
e. all of the answers are correct

16. High doses of digestive enzymes may produce _____ as an adverse effect.

a. nausea
b. diarrhea
c. rash
d. answers a and b are correct
e. answers b and c are correct

17. Digestive enzymes may _____ .

a. be taken before or with meals in a capsule form
b. be sprinkled on soft foods
c. not be chewed if in the time-released capsule form
d. cause nausea and diarrhea
e. all of the answers are correct

18. A patient who has ingested a corrosive substance _____ .

a. should be given an emetic immediately
b. should be told to eat digestive enzymes
c. should not be given an emetic
d. answers a and b are correct
e. none of the answers are correct

19. Gallstone-solubilizing drugs may _____ .

a. suppress the production of cholesterol and cholic acid by the liver
b. be used cautiously during pregnancy
c. be effective for all types of gallstones
d. rarely produce adverse reactions
e. answers a and b are correct

20. A patient who has had a recent myocardial infarction and should not strain during defecation may be given _____ as a laxative.

a. mineral oil
b. saline
c. bulk-producing products
d. hyperosmotic agents
e. a stimulant or irritant

21. A "laxative habit" can result from _____ .

a. an electrolyte imbalance
b. prolonged use of a laxative
c. diarrhea
d. multiple types of laxatives being used for a short time
e. none of the answers are correct

22. Which of the following laxatives is not a Pregnancy Category C drug?

a. cascara
b. mineral oil
c. sagrada

d. docusate
e. phenolphthalein

23. Pantoprazole and rabeprazole are examples of _____ .
   a. laxatives
   b. emetics
   c. proton pump inhibitors
   d. digestive enzymes
   e. gastrointestinal stimulants

24. Olsalazine can be used to treat _____ .
   a. ulcerative colitis
   b. duodenal ulcers
   c. peptic ulcers
   d. chronic inflammatory bowel disease
   e. constipation

25. _____ can be used to treat Crohn's disease.
   a. Sucralfate
   b. Olsalazine
   c. Mesalamine
   d. Sulfasalazine
   e. Misoprostol

26. Patients should consult their physician before using chamomile products if they are being treated with _____ .
   a. warfarin
   b. ardeparin
   c. danaparoid
   d. enoxaparin
   e. all of the answers are correct

27. Chamomile has been used to _____ .
   a. reduce flatulence caused by a nervous stomach
   b. treat the common cold
   c. increase appetite
   d. relieve menstrual cramps
   e. all of the answers are correct

XI. RECALL FACTS

Indicate which of the following statements are Facts with an F. If the statement is not a fact, leave the line blank.

About Interactions of Miscellaneous Gastrointestinal Drugs

_____ 1. Misoprostol and magnesium-containing antacids used concurrently increase the risk of diarrhea.

_____ 2. Iron absorption increases with sulfasalazine use.

_____ 3. Salicylate toxicity is not a risk for patients taking aspirin-containing drugs and bismuth subsalicylate concurrently.

_____ 4. Sulfasalazine and methenamine taken concurrently increase the risk of crystalluria.

_____ 5. Toxicity risk for patients taking sulfasalazine concurrently with oral hypoglycemic drugs increases.

About Patient Management Issues with Drugs That Affect the Gastrointestinal System

_____ 1. Antacids should not be given within 2 hours before or after administration of other oral drugs.

_____ 2. Oral metoclopramide should be given 30 minutes after each meal.

_____ 3. Emetics are the drug of choice for all ingested poisons.

_____ 4. Mineral oil should be given in the evening on an empty stomach.

_____ 5. Omeprazole should be swallowed whole before taking a meal.

XII. FILL IN THE BLANK

Fill in the blanks using words from the list below.

decreased
dexpanthenol
months
simethicone
digestive enzymes
Robinul
constipation
metoclopramide
histamine H_2
antagonists
pancreatin

urinary retention
medulla
chamomile
decrease
fluids
diarrhea
1–2 hours
pregnancy
duodenal
pancrelipase

1. Calcium-containing antacids may produce _____, whereas sodium-containing antacids can produce _____ .

2. Corticosteroids, digoxin, and chlorpromazine have a(n) _____ pharmacological effect when administered with an antacid.

3. _____ is an example of an anticholinergic drug used for gastrointestinal tract disorders.

4. _____ is an adverse reaction that may occur during treatment with anticholinergic drugs.

5. Oral preparations of _____ are used to treat gastric stasis.

6. A common adverse reaction to the administration of _____ is intestinal colic, which may occur within 30 minutes of administration.

7. Older adults are particularly sensitive to the effects of _____ .

8. Antidiarrheals _____ intestinal peristalsis.

9. Patients with chronic diarrhea are encouraged to ingest extra _____ .

10. _____ works by dispersing and preventing gas pockets in the intestine.

11. _____ and _____ break down and help digest fats, starches, and proteins in food.

12. Patients who have a hypersensitivity to hog or cow proteins should not take _____ .

13. Emetics are used to cause vomiting by stimulating the _____ .

14. Ursodiol may require many _____ of use before results are noted.

15. Proton pump inhibitors are an important part of the treatment of _____ caused by *Helicobacter pylori*.

16. No oral drugs should be given within _____ of an antacid.

17. Ginger is not recommended for morning sickness associated with _____ .

18. _____ may produce symptoms ranging from contact dermatitis to severe anaphylactic reactions in persons hypersensitive to ragweed, asters, and chrysanthemums.

XIII. LIST

List the requested number of items.

1. List six agents used to treat *Helicobacter pylori*.

   a. _____
   b. _____
   c. _____
   d. _____
   e. _____
   f. _____

2. List six types of laxatives.

   a. _____
   b. _____
   c. _____
   d. _____
   e. _____
   f. _____

3. List the three ways that antacids may interfere with other drugs.

   a. _____
   b. _____
   c. _____

4. List four conditions in which histamine H_2 antagonists are used for treatment.

   a. _____
   b. _____
   c. _____
   d. _____

5. List six conditions or diseases for which digestive enzymes may be prescribed.

a. _____

b. _____

c. _____

d. _____

e. _____

f. _____

6. List three common adverse reactions of proton pump inhibitors.

a. _____

b. _____

c. _____

7. List five reasons ginger may be used.

a. _____

b. _____

c. _____

d. _____

e. _____

XIV. CLINICAL APPLICATION

1. Mr. K has been diagnosed with a duodenal ulcer caused by *Helicobacter pylori*. His healthcare provider has decided that the best option for treatment is the combination drug Helidac. Explain to Mr. K how and when to take the various drugs in the dose regimen.

22 | Antidiabetic Drugs

I. MATCHING

Match the term from Column A with the correct definition from Column B.

COLUMN A

_____ 1. diabetes mellitus

_____ 2. diabetic ketoacidosis

_____ 3. glucagon

_____ 4. hyperglycemia

_____ 5. hypoglycemia

_____ 6. lipodystrophy

_____ 7. insulin

COLUMN B

A. Low blood glucose level.
B. Elevated blood glucose level.
C. A potentially life-threatening deficiency of insulin.
D. Atrophy of subcutaneous fat.
E. A hormone produced by the alpha cells of the pancreas that increases blood sugar by stimulating the conversion of glycogen to glucose in the liver.
F. A chronic disorder characterized by either insufficient insulin production in the beta cells of the pancreas or by cellular resistance to insulin.
G. A hormone produced by the pancreas that helps maintain blood glucose levels within normal limits.

II. MATCHING

Match the generic name of insulin in Column A with the type of insulin in Column B. You may use an answer more than once.

COLUMN A

_____ 1. insulin zinc suspension

_____ 2. insulin lispro

_____ 3. insulin injection (regular)

_____ 4. insulin glargine solution

_____ 5. extended insulin zinc suspension

_____ 6. insulin aspart solution

_____ 7. insulin injection concentrate

_____ 8. isophane insulin suspension and insulin inject (NPH)

COLUMN B

A. Rapid-acting
B. Intermediate-acting
C. Long-acting
D. Mixed insulin
E. High-potency insulin

III. MATCHING

Match the generic antidiabetic drug in Column A with the correct trade name in Column B.

COLUMN A

_____ 1. glimepiride

_____ 2. nateglinide

_____ 3. miglitol

_____ 4. glyburide

_____ 5. acetohexamide

_____ 6. chlorpropamide

_____ 7. acarbose

_____ 8. tolazamide

_____ 9. metformin

_____ 10. glipizide

_____ 11. pioglitazone HCl

_____ 12. tolbutamide

_____ 13. glyburide/metformin HCl

_____ 14. rosiglitazone

COLUMN B

A. DiaBeta
B. Orinase
C. Tolinase
D. Starlix
E. Amaryl
F. Glyset
G. Diabinese
H. Glucotrol
I. Precose
J. Glucophage
K. Dymelor
L. Avandia
M. Glucovance
N. Actos

IV. MATCHING

Match the antidiabetic drug in Column A with the type of drug in Column B. You may use an answer more than once.

COLUMN A

_____ 1. Dymelor

_____ 2. Prandin

_____ 3. Amaryl

_____ 4. Glyset

_____ 5. Glucovance

_____ 6. Micronase

_____ 7. Glucophage

_____ 8. Actos

_____ 9. Orinase

_____ 10. Precose

COLUMN B

A. Sulfonylurea
B. Alpha-glucosidase inhibitor
C. Biguanide
D. Meglitinide
E. Thiazolidinediones
F. Antidiabetic combination drug

V. TRUE/FALSE

Indicate whether each statement is True (T) or False (F).

_____ 1. Proglycem is an antidiabetic combination drug.

_____ 2. Diabetes mellitus is treated with the same drugs as diabetes insipidus.

_____ 3. Type 1 diabetics are often treated with oral hypoglycemics.

_____ 4. Type 2 diabetes is easier to control than type 1 diabetes.

_____ 5. Human insulin is derived from a biosynthetic process using strains of *Escherichia coli*.

_____ 6. Human insulin appears to cause fewer allergic reactions than insulin from animal sources.

_____ 7. Hyperglycemia may occur if there is too little insulin in the bloodstream in relation to the available glucose.

_____ 8. Hypoglycemic reactions are most likely to occur when insulin is at its peak activity.

_____ 9. Animal-based insulin products produce fewer hypoglycemic symptoms than do human insulin products.

_____ 10. There is no standard dose of insulin.

_____ 11. Insulin can be administered by any route.

_____ 12. Lipodystrophy can interfere with the absorption of insulin from the injection site.

_____ 13. Diabetic ketoacidosis results in hyperglycemia caused by a deficiency of insulin.

_____ 14. Some patients with diabetes can be noncompliant.

_____ 15. Miglitol is an example of a meglitinide antidiabetic drug.

_____ 16. Sulfonylureas act by stimulating the beta cells of the pancreas to release insulin.

_____ 17. Metformin is the only biguanide type antidiabetic drug.

_____ 18. Meglitinides act by stimulating the release of insulin from the beta cells of the pancreas.

_____ 19. Starlix is an alpha glucosidase inhibitor type of antidiabetic drug.

_____ 20. Repaglinide is an example of a thiazolidinedione.

_____ 21. Oral antidiabetic drugs can be used by either type 1 or type 2 diabetics with equal success.

_____ 22. Adverse reactions of sulfonylureas may be reduced or eliminated by changing the dosage or giving the drug in divided doses.

_____ 23. Lactic acidosis may occur with metformin use.

_____ 24. The most common adverse reactions of alpha glucosidase inhibitors are bloating and flatulence.

_____ 25. The alpha glucosidase inhibitors are considered to be Pregnancy Category B drugs.

_____ 26. Meglitinides are safe to use in patients with type 1 diabetes.

_____ 27. Repaglinide is safe to use during pregnancy and lactation.

_____ 28. There is no fixed dosage for the treatment of diabetes.

_____ 29. A patient who is stabilized with an oral antidiabetic drug but who undergoes a stressful event may require insulin.

_____ 30. Acarbose and miglitol are given three times a day with the first bite of the meal.

VI. MULTIPLE CHOICE

Circle the letter of the best answer.

1. Which of the following is a glucose-elevating drug?
   a. repaglinide
   b. glucagons
   c. Glucovance
   d. glyburide
   e. Diabinese

2. Which of the following antidiabetic drugs is used as an adjunct to diet to lower blood glucose in type 2 diabetes?
   a. nateglinide
   b. NovoLog
   c. chlorpropamide
   d. diazoxide
   e. Lantus

3. Patients with diabetes mellitus can _____ .
   a. produce too much insulin
   b. produce too little insulin
   c. have cells hypersensitive to insulin
   d. have cells resistant to insulin
   e. answers b and d are correct

4. Major adverse reactions seen with insulin administration are _____ .
   a. hypoglycemia
   b. antibody development to insulin
   c. hyperglycemia
   d. allergic reactions
   e. all of the answers are correct

5. Insulin would be contraindicated in which of the following patients?
   a. a hypoglycemic patient
   b. a hyperglycemic patient
   c. a patient hypersensitive to product ingredients
   d. a lactating woman
   e. answers a and c are correct

6. Insulin may be injected into which of the following sites?
   a. arms
   b. thighs
   c. abdomen
   d. buttocks
   e. all of the answers are correct

7. Insulin is absorbed most rapidly in the _____ .
   a. upper arm
   b. abdomen
   c. thigh
   d. buttocks
   e. all sites absorb insulin equally well

8. Which of the following is not a type of oral antidiabetic drug?
   a. sulfonylureas
   b. sulfonamides
   c. biguanides
   d. meglitinides
   e. thiazolidinediones

9. Which of the following drugs is an example of an alpha glucosidase inhibitor?
   a. glyburide
   b. metformin
   c. nateglinide
   d. miglitol
   e. pioglitazone

10. _____ is an example of a biguanide.
    a. Metformin
    b. Repaglinide
    c. Glimepiride

d. Acarbose

e. Rosiglitazone

11. Which of the following drugs is not a second- or third-generation sulfonylurea?

   a. glimepiride
   b. glyburide
   c. glipizide
   d. tolbutamide
   e. amaryl

12. Biguanides act by _____ .

   a. stimulating the beta cells of the pancreas to produce extra insulin
   b. stimulating the beta cells of the pancreas to release insulin
   c. reducing hepatic glucose production
   d. increasing insulin sensitivity in muscle and fat cells
   e. answers c and d are correct

13. Thiazolidinediones act by _____ .

   a. increasing the release of insulin by the beta cells of the pancreas
   b. decreasing insulin resistance
   c. increasing insulin sensitivity
   d. decreasing insulin sensitivity
   e. answers b and c are correct

14. Oral antidiabetic drugs may be _____ .

   a. used in type 2 diabetics whose diet does not control their condition
   b. used with insulin in some patients
   c. used in combination (i.e., two antidiabetic drugs)
   d. answers a and c are correct
   e. all of the answers are correct

15. Metformin _____ .

   a. is sometimes given to obese diabetic patients to help with weight loss
   b. can decrease vitamin B_{12} levels
   c. can cause lactic acidosis
   d. rarely causes hypoglycemia
   e. all of the answers are correct

16. Patients receiving thiazolidinediones in combination with insulin or other hypoglycemic medications are _____ .

   a. at a decreased risk for hypoglycemia
   b. at an increased risk for hypoglycemia
   c. at an increased risk for hyperglycemia
   d. at a decreased risk for hyperglycemia
   e. answers a and c are correct

17. Metformin is contraindicated in all the following patients except _____ .

   a. those older than 80 years of age
   b. those who are pregnant or lactating
   c. those using NSAIDs
   d. those with heart failure
   e. those with acute or chronic metabolic acidosis

18. The effects of acarbose may increase when used with all of the following drugs except _____ .

   a. digestive enzymes
   b. loop or thiazide diuretics
   c. glucocorticoids
   d. oral contraceptives
   e. calcium channel blockers

19. In which of the following conditions are alpha glucosidase inhibitors contraindicated?

   a. cirrhosis
   b. hypersensitivity to the drug
   c. diabetic ketoacidosis
   d. chronic intestinal disease
   e. all of the answers are correct

20. All of the following drugs, when used with a meglitinide, may decrease the hypoglycemic action of the drug except _____ .

   a. thiazides
   b. corticosteroids
   c. thyroid drugs
   d. salicylates
   e. sympathomimetics

21. Which of the following factors are considered when the drug regimen is determined for a diabetic?

   a. effectiveness of the drug
   b. tolerance of the drug
   c. maximum recommended dosage
   d. answers a and c are correct
   e. all of the answers are correct

22. Which of the following sulfonylureas are given 30 minutes before a meal?

   a. glipizide
   b. glyburide
   c. glimepiride
   d. tolbutamide
   e. acetohexamide

23. Secondary failure can occur when _____ .

   a. there is a decreased response to a drug
   b. there is an increase in the severity of the disease

c. the sulfonylurea loses its effectiveness
d. answers a and c are correct
e. all of the answers are correct

24. A patient taking an alpha glucosidase inhibitor has a hypoglycemic reaction. Which of the following should not be given to terminate the reaction?

a. glucose tablets
b. dextrose
c. sugar (sucrose)
d. all of the answers are correct
e. none of the answers are correct

VII. RECALL FACTS

Indicate which of the following statements are Facts with an F. If the statement is not a fact, leave the line blank.

About Products That May Increase the Hypoglycemic Effect of Insulin

_____ 1. alcohol

_____ 2. diuretics

_____ 3. calcium

_____ 4. estrogen

_____ 5. salicylates

_____ 6. clonidine

_____ 7. niacin

_____ 8. tetracycline

About Products That May Decrease the Hypoglycemic Effect of Insulin

_____ 1. MAOIs

_____ 2. oral contraceptives

_____ 3. corticosteroids

_____ 4. ACE inhibitors

_____ 5. epinephrine

_____ 6. beta blocking drugs

_____ 7. thyroid hormones

_____ 8. albuterol

About Drugs with Which Sulfonylureas Will Have an Increased Hypoglycemic Effect

_____ 1. anticoagulants

_____ 2. corticosteroids

_____ 3. histamine H_2 antagonists

_____ 4. clofibrate

_____ 5. calcium channel blockers

_____ 6. estrogen

_____ 7. salicylates

_____ 8. MAOIs

VIII. FILL IN THE BLANK

Fill in the blanks using words from the list below.

recombinant DNA	acarbose
hypoglycemia	ketones
milk production	increase
subcutaneously	immediately
decrease	type 1 diabetes
glucometer	glitazones
glucose	hypoglycemia
oral antidiabetic	initial
increased	increase
miglitol	Glucophage XR
oral anticoagulants	glimepiride
metallic taste	fats
coronary artery disease	

1. Insulin analogs, insulin lispro, and insulin aspart are made by using _____ technology.

2. _____ may occur when there is too much insulin in the bloodstream in relation to the available glucose.

3. Insulin appears to inhibit _____.

4. A diabetic who is pregnant should expect her insulin requirement to _____ in the first trimester, _____ in the second and third trimester, but decrease rapidly after delivery.

5. Insulin must be given by the parenteral route, usually _____ .

6. A _____ is a device used to monitor blood glucose levels.

7. Diabetic ketoacidosis results in dangerously high levels of _____ in the blood, which leads the body to begin to break down _____, which when broken down results in _____ being produced by the liver.

8. _____ drugs are used to treat patients with type 2 diabetes but are not effective for treating _____ .

9. _____ and _____ are examples of alpha glucosidase inhibitors.

10. Thiazolidinediones are also called _____.

11. Biguanides can have an adverse reaction of a _____ .

12. Alpha glucosidase inhibitors _____ the transit time of food in the digestive tract.

13. Acarbose and miglitol, when used alone, do not cause _____ .

14. First-generation sulfonylureas are contraindicated in patients with _____ or liver/kidney dysfunction.

15. There is a(n) _____ risk of lactic acidosis when metformin is used with glucocorticoids.

16. Thiazolidinediones may alter the effects of _____ .

17. Patients receiving both insulin and an oral hypoglycemic are observed often during the _____ period of therapy.

18. _____ is given once daily with the first main meal of the day.

19. _____ is given once daily with the evening meal.

20. A hypoglycemic reaction must be terminated _____ .

IX. LIST

List the requested number of items.

1. List three drugs (trade names) used as an adjunct to diet to lower blood glucose levels in type 2 diabetes.

   a. _____

   b. _____

   c. _____

2. List five risk factors for type 2 diabetes.

   a. _____

   b. _____

   c. _____

   d. _____

   e. _____

3. List three functions of insulin.

   a. _____

   b. _____

   c. _____

4. List five uses of insulin.

   a. _____

   b. _____

   c. _____

   d. _____

   e. _____

5. List five methods of ending a hypoglycemic reaction.

   a. _____

   b. _____

   c. _____

   d. _____

   e. _____

6. List six items that should be checked on the physical assessment before the first dose of insulin is given to a recently diagnosed patient with diabetes mellitus.

   a. _____

   b. _____

   c. _____

   d. _____

   e. _____

   f. _____

7. List six signs of hyperglycemia.

   a. _____

   b. _____

   c. _____

   d. _____

   e. _____

   f. _____

8. List five types of antidiabetic drugs.

   a. _____

   b. _____

   c. _____

   d. _____

   e. _____

9. List five adverse reactions of sulfonylureas.

   a. _____

   b. _____

   c. _____

   d. _____

   e. _____

10. List the three first-generation sulfonylureas.

    a. _____

    b. _____

    c. _____

11. List five drugs that increase a patient's risk of hypoglycemia when used with metformin.

    a. _____

    b. _____

    c. _____

    d. _____

    e. _____

X. CLINICAL APPLICATIONS

1. Your neighbor suspects that her son may have type 1 diabetes. What can you tell her about this disorder?

2. You suspect that a diabetic patient who just received their insulin shot is having a hypoglycemic reaction. What symptoms would you expect this patient to exhibit?

23 Hormones and Related Drugs

I. MATCHING

Match the term from Column A with the correct definition from Column B.

COLUMN A

_____ 1. androgens

_____ 2. corticosteroids

_____ 3. diabetes insipidus

_____ 4. estrogens

_____ 5. euthyroid

_____ 6. glucocorticoids

_____ 7. gonadotropins

_____ 8. hyperstimulation syndrome

_____ 9. myxedema

_____ 10. somatotropic hormone

_____ 11. thyroid storm

_____ 12. thyrotoxicosis

COLUMN B

A. The collective name for the glucocorticoids and mineralocorticoids.
B. Hormones that stimulate activity of the accessory male sex organs.
C. Sudden ovarian enlargement with accumulation of serous fluid in the peritoneal cavity.
D. A normal thyroid.
E. A severe form of hyperthyroidism also known as thyrotoxicosis.
F. A growth hormone secreted by the anterior pituitary.
G. A severe form of hyperthyroidism, also known as thyroid storm.
H. Hormones that promote growth and function of the gonads.
I. A hormone essential to life produced by the adrenal cortex.
J. A severe hypothyroidism manifested by a variety of symptoms.
K. Female hormones influenced by the anterior pituitary gland.

L. A disease resulting from the failure of the posterior pituitary to secrete vasopressin or from surgical removal of the pituitary.

II. MATCHING

Match the generic drug name in Column A with the type of hormone or production site in Column B. You may use an answer more than once.

COLUMN A

_____ 1. fludrocortisone acetate

_____ 2. liotrix

_____ 3. menotropins

_____ 4. betamethasone

_____ 5. triamcinolone

_____ 6. fluoxymesterone

_____ 7. estradiol hemihydrate

_____ 8. norethindrone acetate

_____ 9. levothyroxine sodium

_____ 10. desmopressin acetate

_____ 11. testosterone enanthate

_____ 12. clomiphene citrate

_____ 13. estropipate

_____ 14. dexamethasone

_____ 15. somatrem

_____ 16. vasopressin

COLUMN B

A. Anterior pituitary
B. Posterior pituitary
C. Glucocorticoids
D. Mineralocorticoids
E. Thyroid hormones
F. Androgens
G. Estrogens
H. Progestins

III. MATCHING

Match the generic drug name in Column A with the correct trade name in Column B.

COLUMN A

_____ 1. testosterone enanthate

_____ 2. medroxyprogesterone acetate

_____ 3. clomiphene citrate

_____ 4. conjugated estrogens

_____ 5. urofollitropin

_____ 6. prednisolone

_____ 7. corticotrophin

_____ 8. liotrix

_____ 9. lypressin

_____ 10. triamcinolone acetonide

_____ 11. menotropins

_____ 12. estradiol, oral

_____ 13. dexamethasone

_____ 14. methimazole

_____ 15. hydrocortisone

_____ 16. betamethasone

COLUMN B

A. Diapid
B. Cortef
C. Acthar
D. Decadron
E. Fertinex
F. Thyrolar
G. Celestone
H. Prelone
I. Delastryl
J. Kenalog-10
K. Clomid
L. Premarin
M. Tapazole
N. Estrace
O. Depo-Provera
P. Pergonal

IV. MATCHING

Match the trade name in Column A with the correct use in Column B. You may use an answer more than once.

COLUMN A

_____ 1. Android

_____ 2. Tapazole

_____ 3. Premarin

_____ 4. Protropin

_____ 5. Halotestin

_____ 6. Amen

_____ 7. Diapid

_____ 8. Humegon

_____ 9. Cytomel

_____ 10. Menest

_____ 11. Eltroxin

_____ 12. Clomid

_____ 13. Stimate

_____ 14. Aygestin

_____ 15. Genotropin

COLUMN B

A. Ovulatory failure
B. Growth failure
C. Diabetes insipidus
D. Hypothyroidism
E. Hyperthyroidism
F. Inoperable breast cancer
G. Vasomotor symptoms
H. Amenorrhea
I. Male hypogonadism

V. MATCHING

Match the trade name of the drug in Column A with the type of drug in Column B. You may use an answer more than once.

COLUMN A

_____ 1. PTU

_____ 2. Deca-Durabolin

_____ 3. Thyro-Block

_____ 4. Iodotope

_____ 5. Cortifoam

_____ 6. Oxandrin

_____ 7. Tapazole

_____ 8. Anadrol-50

_____ 9. Proscar

_____ 10. Winstrol

COLUMN B

A. Corticosteroid retention enemas
B. Antithyroid preps
C. Iodine products
D. Anabolic steroids
E. Androgen hormone inhibitors

VI. TRUE/FALSE

Indicate whether each statement is True (T) or False (F).

_____ 1. Pergonal and Metrodin are purified preparations extracted from the urine of postmenopausal women.

_____ 2. Multiple births and birth defects have been reported with the use of both menotropin and urofollitropin.

_____ 3. Urofollitropin can produce adverse reactions of hemoperitoneum and febrile reactions.

_____ 4. Metrodin is contraindicated during pregnancy.

_____ 5. There are many clinically significant interactions with the gonadotropins.

_____ 6. Gonadotropin drugs are destroyed by the gastrointestinal tract so must be given intramuscularly.

_____ 7. Somatotropic hormone may be given to children of any age regardless of epiphyseal closure.

_____ 8. Growth hormones cause few adverse reactions when administered as directed.

_____ 9. Corticotropin stimulates the anterior pituitary to produce glucocorticoids.

_____ 10. Patients taking corticotropins should avoid any vaccinations with live viruses.

_____ 11. Clomiphene therapy may be continued for up to 8 months before the drug is considered unsuccessful.

_____ 12. Lypressin and desmopressin are derivatives of vasopressin.

_____ 13. Vasopressin is contraindicated in patients who have an allergy to pork or pork proteins.

_____ 14. Older patients are less sensitive to the effects of vasopressin because of their decreased kidney function.

_____ 15. Examples of mineralocorticoids are cortisone and prednisone.

_____ 16. When a serious disease is being treated with glucocorticoids, the appearance of Cushing-like symptoms indicates that the drug should be immediately discontinued.

_____ 17. Death can result from circulatory collapse if adrenal insufficiency is not treated promptly.

_____ 18. Florinef is the only currently available mineralocorticoid drug.

_____ 19. Patients with systemic fungal infections should not receive fludrocortisone.

_____ 20. A patient receiving a short-acting glucocorticoid on alternate days before 9 AM will have a greater response because of the release of additional endogenous hormone later in the day.

_____ 21. The most common adverse reactions of thyroid hormone therapy are signs of overdose and hyperthyroidism.

_____ 22. Older adults are more likely to experience adverse reactions to thyroid replacement therapy.

_____ 23. Radioactive iodine is used to treat hypothyroidism.

_____ 24. Generally speaking, synthetic thyroid hormones are preferred medically because they are more uniform in potency than natural hormones.

_____ 25. Levothyroxine is the drug of choice for hypothyroidism.

_____ 26. For best results, thyroid hormones should be administered once-a-day, early in the morning, and on an empty stomach.

_____ 27. Synthroid is only given as an oral preparation.

_____ 28. The therapeutic effects of antithyroid drugs are seen immediately since they neutralize existing thyroid hormones in circulation and storage.

_____ 29. An oral solution of Lugol's may be given to a patient to help prepare them for thyroid surgery.

_____ 30. Iodine solutions should be drunk through a straw to avoid tooth discoloration.

_____ 31. Virilization is one of the most common adverse reactions in women receiving an androgen preparation for breast cancer.

_____ 32. Illegal use of anabolic steroids in young, healthy individuals has resulted in deaths.

_____ 33. Prolonged high-dose anabolic steroid use can become psychologically and possibly physically addicting.

_____ 34. Older men treated with anabolic steroids are at no higher risk for prostatic enlargement and prostate cancer than younger men.

_____ 35. Proscar use results in a decrease in the size of the prostate gland and therefore is used to treat the symptoms of benign prostatic hypertrophy.

_____ 36. Adverse reactions to finasteride are usually mild and do not require discontinuation of the drug.

_____ 37. Anabolic steroid or androgen use by older adults with cardiac problems or kidney disease results in an increased risk for sodium and water retention.

_____ 38. Synthetic progestins are preferred for medical use.

_____ 39. Estrogens have few adverse reactions when given by the correct route.

_____ 40. The use of a levonorgestrel implant system may result in hyperpigmentation at the implant site.

_____ 41. Cigarette smoking increases the risk for cardiovascular complications in patients receiving estrogen therapy.

_____ 42. Oral estrogens are administered with food or immediately after eating to reduce gastrointestinal upset.

_____ 43. The Norplant system is a combination estrogen/progestin contraceptive which when implanted provides 5 years of protection.

_____ 44. Medroxyprogesterone acetate is used in the treatment of abnormal uterine bleeding, secondary amenorrhea, and as a contraceptive.

_____ 45. Black cohosh is thought to increase diminished estrogen levels in menopausal women.

_____ 46. Saw palmetto is most active when taken in the tea form.

VII. MULTIPLE CHOICE

Circle the letter of the best answer.

1. Menotropins, when given to men, induce _____ .
   a. the release of testosterone
   b. the production of sperm
   c. the inhibition of androgen release
   d. the production of prostatic secretions
   e. the male secondary sex characteristics to appear

2. _____ is used to induce ovulation in women with polycystic ovarian disease.
   a. Menotropin
   b. Pergonal
   c. Metrodin
   d. Urofollitropin
   e. Answers c and d are correct

3. _____ is a synthetic, nonsteroidal compound that binds to estrogen receptors, which results in an increased secretion of follicle-stimulating hormone and luteinizing hormone.
   a. Pergonal
   b. Metrodin
   c. Clomid
   d. Protropin
   e. Humatrope

4. Clomiphene and chorionic gonadotrophin are used to _____ .
   a. treat prepubertal cryptorchism
   b. induce ovulation in anovulatory women
   c. treat hypogonadotropic hypogonadism
   d. treat polycystic ovaries
   e. reduce scrotal development

5. Chorionic gonadotropin administration is contraindicated in all of the following patients except a patient with _____ .
   a. liver disease
   b. precocious puberty
   c. prostatic cancer
   d. pregnancy
   e. androgen-dependent neoplasm

6. If a patient taking clomiphene complains of _____, the drug is discontinued and the healthcare provider is notified.
   a. ovarian stimulation or enlargement
   b. asthma
   c. migraine headaches
   d. visual disturbances
   e. answers a and d are correct

7. In hyperstimulation syndrome, the patient may present with which of the following indicators?
   a. anxiety
   b. abdominal pain and distention
   c. redness and irritation at the injection site
   d. epilepsy
   e. renal dysfunction

8. Corticotropin is used with caution in children because it can _____ .
   a. cause scleroderma
   b. decrease the need for insulin in diabetics
   c. inhibit skeletal growth
   d. cause congestive heart failure
   e. alter kidney function

9. A patient receiving prolonged corticotrophin therapy should be monitored for _____ changes.
   a. liver
   b. hematological, electrolyte, and glucose
   c. cardiovascular
   d. reproductive system
   e. respiratory system

10. Vasopressin therapy may be used to _____ .
    a. treat diabetes insipidus
    b. prevent and treat postoperative abdominal distention
    c. dispel gas that interferes with abdominal radiographs
    d. answers b and c are correct
    e. all of the answers are correct

11. Pitressin Synthetic is the trade name for _____ .
    a. lypressin
    b. oxytocin

c. vasopressin
d. desmopressin
e. Diapid

12. The antidiuretic effect of vasopressin may be increased when taken with _____ .
    a. carbamazepine
    b. alcohol
    c. heparin
    d. lithium
    e. norepinephrine

13. When being treated with vasopressin the patient _____ .
    a. may drink alcohol
    b. should measure the amount of fluids drunk each day
    c. should drink one or two glasses of water immediately after taking the drug
    d. should use the same injection site repeatedly
    e. answers a and c are correct

14. When discontinuing glucocorticoid therapy _____ .
    a. the dosage must be tapered off over several days
    b. the dosage may be abruptly discontinued to prompt the adrenal glands to function again
    c. no tapering is required when therapy extends beyond 5 days
    d. answers b and c are correct
    e. none of the answers are correct—glucocorticoid therapy is never discontinued

15. Adverse reactions, in addition to adrenal insufficiency, that are associated with glucocorticoid therapy may include all of the following except _____ .
    a. peptic ulcers
    b. fractures
    c. infection
    d. fluid and electrolyte imbalance
    e. malabsorption syndrome

16. Glucocorticoids are contraindicated in which of the following conditions?
    a. renal disease
    b. serious infections
    c. ulcerative colitis
    d. diabetes mellitus
    e. pregnancy

17. Fludrocortisone _____ .
    a. has mineralocorticoid activity
    b. has glucocorticoid activity
    c. is used for replacement therapy for primary adrenocortical deficiency
    d. is used for replacement therapy for secondary adrenocortical deficiency
    e. all of the answers are correct

18. Mrs. P is receiving corticosteroid therapy and should be monitored regularly for which of the following?
    a. blood pressure
    b. signs of infection
    c. electrolyte imbalance
    d. mental status
    e. all of the answers are correct

19. Alternate-day administration of glucocorticoids _____ .
    a. gives the patient a day of medicinal rest
    b. provides the patient with the beneficial effects of the drug while minimizing certain undesirable reactions
    c. allows the drug to be fully metabolized before the next dose
    d. keeps the anterior pituitary gland from being activated
    e. none of the answers are correct

20. Plasma levels of endogenous adrenocortical hormones are normally higher _____ .
    a. between 4 PM and midnight
    b. between 8 AM and 4 PM
    c. between 2 AM and 8 AM
    d. after strenuous exercise
    e. every other day

21. Synthroid is the drug of choice for hypothyroidism for all of the following reasons except that it _____ .
    a. is relatively inexpensive
    b. is difficult for the patient to manage
    c. requires once-a-day dosing
    d. has a more uniform potency than other drugs
    e. is a synthetic form of the hormone

22. Which of the following are signs of hyperthyroidism?
    a. flushed, warm, moist skin
    b. moderate hypertension
    c. tachycardia
    d. elevated body temperature
    e. all of the answers are correct

23. In which of the following patients are thyroid hormones contraindicated?
    a. pregnant women
    b. lactating women
    c. after recent myocardial infarction
    d. Addison's disease
    e. elderly men

24. A patient receiving thyroid hormones may experience a decreased effectiveness of _____ .
    a. digitalis
    b. oral anticoagulants
    c. oral contraceptives
    d. antacids
    e. live vaccines

25. Drugs used for the medical management of hyperthyroidism include _____ .
    a. propylthiouracil
    b. Tapazole
    c. PTU
    d. methimazole
    e. all of the answers are correct

26. Patients taking antithyroid drugs should be monitored for _____ .
    a. signs of infection
    b. hypercoagulation
    c. liver dysfunction
    d. visual disturbances
    e. ototoxicity

27. When iodine solutions are administered, the patient should be closely monitored for symptoms of _____ .
    a. iodism
    b. swelling around the mouth
    c. difficulty breathing
    d. iodine allergy
    e. all of the answers are correct

28. Radioactive iodine _____ .
    a. is given orally as a single dose
    b. effects occur within 24 hours
    c. requires the patient to remain inactive
    d. frequently causes a thyroid storm to occur
    e. answers a and b are correct

29. Androgen therapy in males is used for _____ .
    a. treatment of hypergonadism
    b. replacement therapy for testosterone deficiency
    c. treatment of precocious puberty
    d. inhibition of testicular development
    e. as part of a treatment regimen in men who have prostatic tumors

30. Adverse reactions of males to androgen therapy may include which of the following?

    a. fluid and electrolyte imbalances
    b. virilization
    c. hair regrowth
    d. clearing of acne
    e. testicular enlargement

31. Anabolic steroids work by _____ .

    a. decreasing endogenous production of androgens
    b. imitating the action of glucocorticoids
    c. stimulating androgen release
    d. promoting tissue building processes
    e. blocking the action of estrogen

32. Proscar _____ .

    a. is a synthetic compound drug
    b. is an androgen hormone inhibitor
    c. has a generic name of finasteride
    d. inhibits the conversion of testosterone into 5 alpha-dihydrotestosterone
    e. all of the answers are correct

33. An example of a progestin is _____ .

    a. Ortho-Est
    b. Aygestin
    c. Estrace
    d. Proscar
    e. Oreton Methyl

34. Which of the following is not an endogenous estrogen?

    a. estradiol
    b. estriol
    c. estrone
    d. progesterone
    e. answers a and b are correct

35. All of the following are uses for progestins except one. Identify the exception.

    a. inoperable breast cancer
    b. treatment of amenorrhea
    c. treatment of endometriosis
    d. treatment of functional uterine bleeding
    e. oral contraceptives

36. Warnings associated with the use of estrogens include increased risk of _____ .

    a. endometrial cancer
    b. gallbladder disease
    c. hypertension
    d. thromboembolic disease
    e. all of the answers are correct

37. In which of the following conditions are progestins contraindicated?

    a. thromboembolic disorders
    b. pregnancy
    c. cerebral hemorrhage
    d. impaired liver function
    e. all of the answers are correct

38. Combination oral contraceptives have _____ warnings associated with their use as do estrogens and progestins.

    a. increased
    b. the same
    c. decreased
    d. all of the answers are correct
    e. none of the answers are correct

39. Biphasic oral contraceptives _____ .

    a. are administered in a 21-day regimen, then skip 7 days
    b. are taken daily and continuously
    c. have varying progestin amounts throughout the 21-day cycle, whereas the estrogen may vary or stay the same
    d. have an estrogen dose that is constant for 21 days, which is then followed by no estrogen; the progestin dose is small the first 10 days, followed by a larger dose of progestin during the last 10 days
    e. none of the answers are correct

40. Mrs. R forgot to take her oral contraceptive on Tuesday. She then took two doses on Wednesday to make up for the missed dose. Because of this Mrs. R _____ .

    a. has no increased chance of pregnancy
    b. has an increased chance of pregnancy
    c. should discontinue the oral contraceptives for the rest of the month
    d. may require a higher dose to be prescribed next month
    e. answers b and d are correct

41. Black cohosh _____ .

    a. is generally regarded as safe when used as directed
    b. has a primary adverse effect of nausea
    c. should not be taken by pregnant women
    d. may reduce physical and psychological symptoms associated with menopause
    e. all of the answers are correct

42. Saw palmetto often takes _____ of treatment before an improvement in symptoms occurs.
    a. 3–5 days
    b. 1–2 weeks
    c. 1–3 months
    d. 6–12 months
    e. more than 18 months

VIII. RECALL FACTS

Indicate which of the following statements are Facts with an F. If the statement is not a fact, leave the line blank.

About Adverse Reactions of Corticotropins

_____ 1. mental depression

_____ 2. hypotension

_____ 3. anorexia

_____ 4. irregular menses or amenorrhea

_____ 5. petechiae and ecchymosis

_____ 6. hirsutism

_____ 7. increased muscular strength

_____ 8. increased susceptibility to infection

_____ 9. night blindness

_____ 10. drowsiness

About Uses of Estrogen

_____ 1. used in combination with progesterones as contraceptives

_____ 2. used in combination with progesterones in hormone replacement therapy in post-menopausal women

_____ 3. female hypergonadism

_____ 4. relieve vasomotor symptoms of menopause

_____ 5. selected cases of inoperable breast carcinoma

_____ 6. palliative treatment for advanced prostatic carcinoma

_____ 7. atrophic vaginitis

_____ 8. osteoporosis in women past menopause

About Adverse Reactions of Progestins

_____ 1. amenorrhea

_____ 2. breakthrough bleeding

_____ 3. melasma

_____ 4. mental stimulation

_____ 5. decrease in acne

_____ 6. edema

_____ 7. spotting

_____ 8. breast enlargement

IX. FILL IN THE BLANK

Fill in the blanks using words from the list below.

infection	benzyl alcohol
urofollitropin	growth hormone
outpatient	pork
intranasal	X
slow	Norplant
never	finasteride
glucose	contraindicated
water intoxication	agranulocytosis
vasopressin	menotropins
estradiol	decreased
chorionic gonadotropin	3
saw palmetto	A
adrenal insufficiency	glucocorticoids
mineralocorticoids	virilization
conserve	balance
thromboembolic	feminizing
potassium	additive
counteracts	iodism
rapid	hyperthyroidism

1. _____ are used to induce ovulation and pregnancy in anovulatory women.

2. _____ is used to stimulate multiple follicular development in ovulatory women for in vitro fertilization.

3. The actions of _____ are identical to those of the pituitary luteinizing hormone.

4. Gonadotropins are almost always administered on a(n) _____ basis.

5. _____ is also called somatotropic hormone.

6. Protropin and Humatrope are contraindicated in patients sensitive to _____ .

7. Corticotropin may mask signs of _____ .

8. Patients who have an allergy to _____ should not be given corticotropins.

9. _____ is secreted by the posterior pituitary gland when body fluids must be conserved.

10. _____ may be indicative of an excessive dosage of vasopressin.

11. Vasopressin, lypressin, and desmopressin may all be administered by the _____ route.

12. _____ is a critical deficiency of the mineralocorticoids and the glucocorticoids.

13. Mental and emotional changes may occur when _____ are administered.

14. Aldosterone and desoxycorticosterone are _____.

15. Mineralocorticoids _____ sodium and increase the excretion of _____ .

16. A glucocorticoid dosage must _____ be omitted.

17. All patients receiving a glucocorticoid should have frequent checks of blood _____ levels.

18. Thyroid hormones are classified as Pregnancy Category _____ drugs and are considered safe to use during pregnancy.

19. Antithyroid drugs or thyroid antagonists are used to treat _____ .

20. _____ is the most serious adverse reaction associated with methimazole and propylthiouracil.

21. Adverse reactions that occur with the use of strong iodine solutions can include symptoms of _____ .

22. Radioactive iodine is _____ during pregnancy and lactation.

23. When methimazole and propylthiouracil are administered with other bone marrow depressants, there can be a(n) _____ effect on the bone marrow.

24. Androgen therapy for women with hormone-dependent malignant breast tumors _____ the effect of estrogen on these tumors.

25. _____ is the most common adverse reaction in women associated with anabolic steroid use.

26. Anabolic steroids are classified as a Pregnancy Category _____ drug.

27. _____ can be used to help prevent male pattern baldness in men with early signs of hair loss.

28. _____ is the most potent estrogen.

29. Adverse reactions of estrogen/progestin combinations as oral contraceptives can be minimized by adjusting the estrogen/progestin _____ .

30. Oral contraceptives should be discontinued at least 4 weeks before a surgical procedure or prolonged immobilization to avoid _____ complications.

31. Male patients taking female hormones as treatment for inoperable prostatic carcinoma should be reassured that _____ effects are usually minimal.

32. The effects of the progestins are _____ when administered with an anticonvulsant, barbiturate, or rifampin.

33. With prostatic carcinoma the response to female hormone therapy may be _____, but with breast carcinoma the response is usually _____.

34. Levonorgestrel is an implant contraceptive also called _____ .

35. Depo-Provera is given intramuscularly every _____ months.

36. _____, an herb, is used to treat benign prostatic hypertrophy.

X. LIST

List the requested number of items.

1. List five patients in whom menotropins are contraindicated.

   a. _____

   b. _____

   c. _____

   d. _____

   e. _____

2. List five adverse reactions associated with clomiphene administration.

   a. _____

   b. _____

   c. _____

   d. _____

   e. _____

3. List five uses of corticotropins.

   a. _____

   b. _____

   c. _____

   d. _____

   e. _____

4. List four drugs that when taken with vasopressin can decrease its antidiuretic effect.

   a. _____

   b. _____

   c. _____

   d. _____

5. List five uses of glucocorticoids.

   a. _____

   b. _____

   c. _____

   d. _____

   e. _____

6. List five adverse reactions of mineralocorticoid therapy.

   a. _____

   b. _____

   c. _____

   d. _____

   e. _____

7. List three reasons for using caution when older patients are being treated with corticosteroids.

   a. _____

   b. _____

   c. _____

8. List four uses of thyroid hormones.

   a. _____

   b. _____

   c. _____

   d. _____

9. List five adverse reactions seen after the administration of radioactive iodine.

   a. _____

   b. _____

   c. _____

   d. _____

   e. _____

10. List four intended uses of anabolic steroids

    a. _____

    b. _____

    c. _____

    d. _____

11. List five actions of estrogens.

    a. _____

    b. _____

    c. _____

    d. _____

    e. _____

12. List the three types of estrogen and progestin oral contraceptives.

    a. _____

    b. _____

    c. _____

13. List four common adverse reactions of female hormones.

   a. _____

   b. _____

   c. _____

   d. _____

14. List five conditions, other than known hypersensitivity, in which estrogen therapy is contraindicated.

   a. _____

   b. _____

   c. _____

   d. _____

   e. _____

XI. CLINICAL APPLICATIONS

1. Miss H has been diagnosed with systemic lupus erythematosus (SLE) and will be receiving short-term glucocorticoid therapy as part of her initial treatment regimen. She has some concerns about how glucocorticoids will help her with this autoimmune disorder, how she should take this medication, and what sorts of adverse reactions she can expect regarding her diabetes mellitus.

2. Mrs. T, age 47, has been diagnosed with Hashimoto's thyroiditis and will soon begin thyroid hormone treatment for this hypothyroid condition. Her healthcare provider has prescribed Synthroid and wants you to go over the signs of hyperthyroidism with Mrs. T. Explain to Mrs. T why she should be concerned about hyperthyroidism when she has hypothyroidism.

I. MATCHING

Match the term from Column A with the correct definition from Column B.

COLUMN A

_____ 1. uterine atony

_____ 2. ergotism

_____ 3. oxytocic drugs

_____ 4. uterine relaxants

_____ 5. oxytocin

COLUMN B

A. An overdose of ergonovine.
B. Used before birth to induce uterine contractions similar to those of normal labor.
C. An endogenous hormone produced by the posterior pituitary gland.
D. Significantly relaxation of the uterine muscle.
E. Drugs used to manage preterm labor by decreasing uterine activity.

II. MATCHING

Match the generic drug in Column A with the correct trade name in Column B.

COLUMN A

_____ 1. methylergonovine

_____ 2. oxytocin

_____ 3. terbutaline

_____ 4. ritodrine

_____ 5. ergonovine maleate

COLUMN B

A. Yutopar
B. Ergotrate
C. Brethaire, Brethine
D. Pitocin, Syntocinon
E. Methergine

III. MATCHING

Match the drug in Column A with the correct use in Column B. You may use an answer more than once.

COLUMN A

_____ 1. Yutopar

_____ 2. Methergine

_____ 3. Pitocin

_____ 4. Brethaire

_____ 5. Ergotrate

COLUMN B

A. Preterm labor
B. Uterine atony and hemorrhage
C. Routine management after delivery of the placenta
D. Antepartum to initiate or improve uterine contractions

IV. MATCHING

Match the use of oxytocin in Column A to its route of administration in Column B. You may use an answer more than once.

COLUMN A

_____ 1. Stimulate milk ejection

_____ 2. Control postpartum bleeding

_____ 3. Starting labor

_____ 4. Produce uterine contractions in third stage of labor

_____ 5. Management of incomplete abortion

COLUMN B

A. IV
B. IM
C. Intranasally

V. TRUE/FALSE

Indicate whether each statement is True (T) or False (F).

_____ 1. An oxytocic drug is used to stimulate the uterus.

_____ 2. Methylergonovine works by decreasing the strength, duration, and frequency of contractions.

_____ 3. Methylergonovine is used to prevent postpartum and postabortal hemorrhage caused by uterine atony.

_____ 4. Abdominal cramping after ergonovine administration indicates that the drug is effective.

_____ 5. Methylergonovine can be used to induce labor.

_____ 6. Ergonovine may be administered IV or IM.

_____ 7. The exact mechanism of action of oxytocin in normal labor is clearly understood.

_____ 8. It is imperative to discontinue the administration of oxytocin when any adverse reactions are reported.

_____ 9. Excessive stimulation of the uterus can result in uterine rupture or uterine hypertonicity.

_____ 10. Uterine relaxants are useful in the management of preterm labor.

_____ 11. Stimulation of beta$_2$ receptors in the uterus inhibits uterine contractions.

_____ 12. Ritodrine is used to manage preterm labor in pregnancies of less than 20 weeks.

_____ 13. Terbutaline is classified as a beta$_2$ adrenergic agonist.

_____ 14. A rare adverse reaction to terbutaline is pulmonary edema.

_____ 15. Fetal and maternal vital signs need to be monitored every 6 hours while the patient is receiving terbutaline.

VI. MULTIPLE CHOICE

Circle the letter of the best answer.

1. Drugs that stimulate the uterus include all but which of the following?

   a. oxytocin
   b. ergonovine
   c. methylergonovine
   d. terbutaline
   e. answers b and d are correct

2. Ergonovine _____ .

   a. increases the strength of uterine contractions
   b. increases the frequency of uterine contractions
   c. increases the duration of uterine contractions
   d. decreases uterine bleeding
   e. all of the answers are correct

3. A patient who is calcium deficient and receiving ergonovine may _____ .

   a. not respond to the drug
   b. respond to the drug if given IV calcium
   c. overrespond to the drug
   d. go into calcium shock
   e. answers a and b are correct

4. In which instance(s) is ergonovine contraindicated?

   a. known hypersensitivity
   b. hypertension
   c. before delivery of the placenta
   d. answers a and b are correct
   e. all of the answers are correct

5. Methylergonovine is contraindicated in all of the following patients except _____ .

   a. hypertension
   b. pre-eclampsia
   c. known hypersensitivity
   d. answers b and c are correct
   e. all of the answers are correct

6. Methylergonovine is usually _____ .

   a. given IM
   b. given after the delivery of the placenta
   c. given at the time the anterior shoulder is delivered
   d. answers a and c are correct
   e. all of the answers are correct

7. Oxytocin may be administered by the _____ route.

   a. intravenous
   b. intranasal
   c. intramuscular
   d. all of the answers are correct
   e. none of the answers are correct; it is given only by the oral route

8. Uterine relaxants _____ .
   a. increase uterine activity
   b. decrease uterine activity
   c. stimulate the let down reflex
   d. act to inhibit oxytocin release
   e. stimulate the release of oxytocin

9. Ritodrine administration can cause _____ .
   a. diarrhea
   b. anorexia
   c. alterations in fetal and maternal heart rates and blood pressure
   d. rash
   e. petechiae

10. Terbutaline is approved by the FDA to be used to _____ .
    a. treat asthma
    b. treat patients with COPD
    c. manage preterm labor
    d. answers a and b are correct
    e. all of the answers are correct

11. Terbutaline is contraindicated in all of the following except _____ .
    a. severe cardiac problems
    b. after the 20th week of pregnancy
    c. digitalis toxicity
    d. hypertension
    e. known hypersensitivity

12. Terbutaline is administered by the _____ route most often.
    a. parenteral, suppository
    b. IV, IM
    c. IM, topical
    d. oral, subcutaneous
    e. none of these are correct

VII. RECALL FACTS

Indicate which of the following statements are Facts with an F. If the statement is not a fact, leave the line blank.

About Adverse Reactions Associated with Ergonovine and Methylergonovine

_____ 1. bradycardia

_____ 2. numb fingers or toes

_____ 3. dizziness

_____ 4. water intoxication

_____ 5. double vision

_____ 6. nausea and vomiting

_____ 7. anorexia

_____ 8. elevated blood pressure

_____ 9. temporary chest pain

_____ 10. red, swollen tongue

About Conditions in Which Oxytocin Is Contraindicated

_____ 1. hypersensitivity

_____ 2. cephalopelvic disproportion

_____ 3. total placenta previa

_____ 4. hypertension

_____ 5. severe toxemia

_____ 6. hypertonic uterus

_____ 7. digitalis toxicity

_____ 8. obstetric emergencies

VIII. FILL IN THE BLANK

Fill in the blanks using words from the list below.

intravenous	short
discontinued	ergotism
before	rare
water intoxication	calcium deficient
after	upright
ritodrine	pulmonary edema
12 hours	investigational

1. Oxytocic drugs are used _____ birth.

2. Ergonovine is given _____ the delivery of the placenta.

3. _____ is an overdosage of ergonovine which in severe cases can result in coma.

4. Patients who are _____ may not respond to ergonovine.

5. When ergotism occurs, ergonovine must be _____ .

6. Methylergonovine is not usually given by the _____ route as it can cause stroke or sudden hypertension.

7. Adverse reactions to intranasally administered oxytocin are _____ .

8. Oxytocin is a _____ acting drug.

9. Intravenous oxytocin can cause _____ because of the anti-diuretic effect of the drug.

10. Intranasally administered oxytocin requires that the patient be in a(n) _____ position.

11. _____ affects beta$_2$ adrenergic receptors of the uterus.

12. Ritodrine and terbutaline can cause a serious adverse reaction of _____ .

13. Terbutaline is primarily used as a bronchodilator; its use in management of premature labor is _____ .

14. Uterine relaxants are generally continued for at least _____ after contractions have stopped.

IX. LIST

List the requested number of items.

1. List the three uses of uterine drugs.

   a. _____

   b. _____

   c. _____

2. List the three drugs that can be used to stimulate the uterus.

   a. _____

   b. _____

   c. _____

3. List four symptoms of ergotism.

   a. _____

   b. _____

   c. _____

   d. _____

4. List the three effects of oxytocin.

   a. _____

   b. _____

   c. _____

5. List five adverse reactions of oxytocin.

   a. _____

   b. _____

   c. _____

   d. _____

   e. _____

6. List six conditions in which ritodrine is contraindicated.

   a. _____

   b. _____

   c. _____

   d. _____

   e. _____

   f. _____

7. List five adverse reactions of terbutaline.

   a. _____

   b. _____

   c. _____

   d. _____

   e. _____

X. CLINICAL APPLICATION

1. Ms. P has premature contractions that are being treated with a uterine relaxant. As a healthcare worker involved in her case, you note that her respiratory rate has reached 22 breaths/min. What should you do in response to this information? What trouble might Ms. P be having, and what might be done to treat this reaction?

25 | Antibacterial Drugs

I. MATCHING

Match the term from Column A with the correct definition from Column B.

COLUMN A

_____ 1. anaerobic

_____ 2. anaphylactoid reaction

_____ 3. antibacterial

_____ 4. anti-infective

_____ 5. bactericidal

_____ 6. bacteriostatic

_____ 7. cross-allergenicity

_____ 8. cross-sensitivity

_____ 9. penicillinase

_____ 10. prophylaxis

_____ 11. Stevens-Johnson syndrome

_____ 12. superinfection

COLUMN B

A. Active against bacteria.

B. Another word for antibacterial; drugs used to treat infections and bacteria.

C. Serious allergic reaction to a drug which initially exhibits reactions easily confused with less severe disorders.

D. Synonymous with cross-allergenicity.

E. An enzyme that inactivates penicillin.

F. Able to live without oxygen.

G. An agent or drug that destroys bacteria.

H. An overgrowth of bacterial or fungal microorganisms not affected by the antibiotic being used for treatment.

I. Allergy to drugs in the same or related group.

J. Prevention.

K. Drugs that slow or retard the multiplication of bacteria.

L. Unusual or exaggerated allergic reaction.

II. MATCHING

Match the generic name of the sulfonamide, penicillin, or cephalosporin in Column A with the correct trade name in Column B.

COLUMN A

_____ 1. mafenide

_____ 2. penicillin G (aqueous)

_____ 3. trimethoprim and sulfamethoxazole

_____ 4. nafcillin

_____ 5. amoxicillin and clavulanate acid

_____ 6. sulfamethizole

_____ 7. cefdinir

_____ 8. penicillin V

_____ 9. cefaclor

_____ 10. sulfasalazine

_____ 11. cefpodoxime

_____ 12. bacampicillin

_____ 13. ceftriaxone

_____ 14. cloxacillin sodium

_____ 15. cephalexin

COLUMN B

A. Bactrim

B. Unipen

C. Spectrobid

D. Thiosulfil Forte

E. Omnicef

F. Sulfamylon

G. Beepen VK

H. Rocephin

I. Azulfidine

J. Cloxapen

K. Keflex

L. Pfizerpen

M. Vantin

N. Ceclor

O. Augmentin

III. MATCHING

Match the generic name of the tetracycline, macrolide or lincosamide in Column A with the correct trade name in Column B.

COLUMN A

_____ 1. demeclocycline

_____ 2. clindamycin

_____ 3. troleandomycin

_____ 4. clarithromycin

_____ 5. dirithromycin

_____ 6. azithromycin

_____ 7. minocycline

_____ 8. doxycycline

_____ 9. lincomycin

_____ 10. erythromycin ethylsuccinate

COLUMN B

A. Biaxin
B. Cleocin
C. Minocin
D. Tao
E. Dynabac
F. Declomycin
G. EryPed
H. Vibramycin
I. Zithromax
J. Lincocin

IV. MATCHING

Match the generic name of the fluoroquinolone or aminoglycoside in Column A with the correct trade name in Column B.

COLUMN A

_____ 1. enoxacin

_____ 2. ofloxacin

_____ 3. ciprofloxacin

_____ 4. amikacin

_____ 5. moxifloxacin

_____ 6. gentamicin

_____ 7. kanamycin

_____ 8. levofloxacin

_____ 9. tobramycin

_____ 10. netilmicin

COLUMN B

A. Levaquin
B. Kantrex
C. Netromycin
D. Nebcin
E. Avelox
F. Garamycin
G. Floxin
H. Cipro
I. Amikin
J. Penetrex

V. MATCHING

Match the trade name of the drug in Column A to the drug category in Column B. You may use an answer more than once.

COLUMN A

_____ 1. Timentin

_____ 2. Gantanol

_____ 3. Keflex

_____ 4. Wycillin

_____ 5. Vibramycin

_____ 6. Augmentin

_____ 7. Ceclor

_____ 8. Septra

_____ 9. Suprax

_____ 10. Bactocill

_____ 11. Zithromax

_____ 12. Silvadene

_____ 13. Pipracil

_____ 14. Cipro

_____ 15. Amikacin

COLUMN B

A. Sulfonamide—single agent
B. Sulfonamide—multiple preparation
C. Miscellaneous sulfonamide preparation
D. Natural penicillin

E. Semi-synthetic penicillin
F. Aminopenicillin
G. Extended-spectrum penicillin
H. First-generation cephalosporin
I. Second-generation cephalosporin
J. Third-generation cephalosporin
K. Tetracycline
L. Macrolide
M. Lincosamide
N. Fluoroquinolone
O. Aminoglycoside

VI. MATCHING

Match the generic name of the antitubercular, leprostatic, or miscellaneous anti-infective in Column A with the correct trade name in Column B.

COLUMN A

_____ 1. aminosalicylate acid

_____ 2. clofazimine

_____ 3. ethambutol

_____ 4. rifabutin

_____ 5. metronidazole

_____ 6. vancomycin

_____ 7. isoniazid

_____ 8. cycloserine

_____ 9. chloramphenicol

_____ 10. linezolid

_____ 11. isoniazid and rifampin

_____ 12. spectinomycin

COLUMN B

A. Lamprene
B. Trobicin
C. Laniazid
D. Chloromycetin
E. Paser
F. Flagyl
G. Zyvox
H. Vancocin
I. Mycobutin
J. Seromycin Pulvules
K. Rifamate
L. Myambutol

VII. MATCHING

Match the trade name in Column A with the drug category in Column B. You may use an answer more than once.

COLUMN A

_____ 1. Capastat sulfate

_____ 2. Protostat

_____ 3. dapsone

_____ 4. INH

_____ 5. Merrem IV

_____ 6. Rifadin

_____ 7. Paser

_____ 8. Trobicin

_____ 9. Zyvox

_____ 10. Lamprene

COLUMN B

A. Antitubercular—primary
B. Antitubercular—second-line
C. Leprostatic
D. Miscellaneous anti-infective

VIII. TRUE/FALSE

Indicate whether each statement is True (T) or False (F).

_____ 1. Penicillins were the first antibiotic drug developed that effectively treated infections.

_____ 2. Sulfasalazine may cause the urine and skin to be an orange-yellow color.

_____ 3. Crystalluria associated with sulfonamide use may be prevented by increasing fluid intake during therapy.

_____ 4. Stevens-Johnson syndrome can be fatal.

_____ 5. Sulfonamides are a Pregnancy Category C drug and therefore are safe to use during any stage of pregnancy.

_____ 6. A patient taking a sulfonamide drug almost always has an active infection.

_____ 7. Older adults generally have fewer complications with sulfonamides than do younger adults.

_____ 8. Cranberry is believed to prevent bacteria from adhering to the wall of the urinary tract.

_____ 9. Cranberries can cure a urinary tract infection.

_____ 10. Natural penicillins have a fairly narrow spectrum of activity.

_____ 11. Beta-lactamase inhibitors are as effective alone as antibiotics.

_____ 12. Penicillins act by preventing bacteria from using a substance that is necessary for the maintenance of the bacteria's outer cell wall.

_____ 13. Penicillins may be bacteriostatic or bactericidal.

_____ 14. The penicillins are the only antibiotics effective in treating viral and fungal infections.

_____ 15. Glossitis and/or stomatitis are adverse reactions sometimes seen with oral penicillin administration.

_____ 16. Patients with an allergy to one penicillin are most likely allergic to all penicillins and have a higher incidence of allergy to the cephalosporins.

_____ 17. Superinfections may occur with the use of any antibiotic and are potentially life-threatening.

_____ 18. Symptoms of candidiasis can include lesions in the mouth or anal/genital itching.

_____ 19. A black, furry tongue may be a sign of a fungal superinfection caused by oral penicillin use.

_____ 20. Penicillin absorption is not affected by food so it may be taken without regard to meals.

_____ 21. Goldenseal is contraindicated during pregnancy and in patients with hypertension.

_____ 22. Cephalosporins are bacteriostatic.

_____ 23. Cephalosporins may be given prophylactically to patients undergoing gastrointestinal or vaginal surgery.

_____ 24. Therapy with cephalosporins may result in bacterial or fungal superinfections.

_____ 25. Frequent liquid stools in patients receiving cephalosporin therapy indicates that the medication is effectively working.

_____ 26. The tetracyclines, macrolides, and lincosamides are considered to be broad-spectrum antibiotics.

_____ 27. Tetracyclines are bactericidal.

_____ 28. Tetracyclines work by inhibiting bacterial protein synthesis.

_____ 29. The tetracyclines may cause a photosensitivity reaction.

_____ 30. Tetracyclines are safe to give during pregnancy.

_____ 31. Macrolides are particularly effective in treating infections of the respiratory and genital tracts.

_____ 32. Macrolides are safe to use as prophylaxis in patients allergic to penicillins.

_____ 33. All of the macrolides cause severe gastrointestinal disturbances.

_____ 34. Macrolides may cause pseudomembranous colitis.

_____ 35. Lincosamides act by inhibiting protein synthesis.

_____ 36. Lincosamides are effective against Gram-positive and Gram-negative microorganisms.

_____ 37. Lincosamides have a high potential for toxicity.

_____ 38. Fluoroquinolones and aminoglycosides were developed in response to increasing microorganism antibiotic drug resistance.

_____ 39. Fluoroquinolones are bacteriostatic.

_____ 40. Cipro is available in ophthalmic form as well as oral.

_____ 41. Lomefloxacin and sparfloxacin can cause a severe photosensitivity reaction.

_____ 42. All fluoroquinolones can cause the rupture of a tendon.

_____ 43. Aminoglycosides are bacteriocidal.

_____ 44. Aminoglycosides inhibit protein synthesis.

_____ 45. Aminoglycosides are primarily used to treat infections caused by Gram-negative microorganisms.

_____ 46. Nephrotoxicity produced by aminoglycosides is irreversible.

_____ 47. Ototoxicity produced by aminoglycoside therapy may occur during drug therapy or after the drug is discontinued.

_____ 48. Aminoglycoside therapy is contraindicated in patients with parkinsonism.

_____ 49. When an aminoglycoside is being used, the patient's respiratory rate must be monitored.

_____ 50. Fluoroquinolones may be given orally, parenterally, or intramuscularly.

_____ 51. Any complaints from a patient receiving fluoroquinolone or aminoglycoside therapy should be reported.

_____ 52. Antitubercular drug therapy can cure a patient with tuberculosis.

_____ 53. Isoniazid is the only bactericidal antitubercular drug.

_____ 54. Antitubercular drugs work by inhibiting bacterial cell wall synthesis.

_____ 55. Vision changes related to ethambutol are usually reversible if the drug is discontinued as soon as symptoms appear.

_____ 56. Hepatitis, a potential adverse reaction of isoniazid therapy, only occurs during treatment.

_____ 57. Rifampin may cause a reddish-orange discoloration of body fluids.

_____ 58. Isoniazid and rifampin used concurrently may result in a higher risk of hepatotoxicity than when either drug is used alone.

_____ 59. Directly observed therapy for treatment of tuberculosis may be necessary to assure compliance with the treatment regimen.

_____ 60. Leprostatic drugs cure leprosy.

_____ 61. Clofazimine and dapsone have no significant drug–drug interactions.

_____ 62. Clofazimine is bactericidal against _Mycobacterium tuberculosis_.

_____ 63. Patients receiving oral chloramphenicol are often hospitalized.

_____ 64. Patients on linezolid may experience severe hypertension if large amounts of food containing tyramine are ingested.

_____ 65. Meropenem is contraindicated in patients allergic to cephalosporins and penicillins.

_____ 66. Flagyl works by lysing the cell wall of susceptible organisms.

_____ 67. Use of NebuPent may result in a metallic taste in the mouth.

_____ 68. Spectinomycin is an aminoglycoside.

_____ 69. Trobicin interferes with bacterial protein synthesis.

_____ 70. Spectinomycin is contraindicated in infants.

_____ 71. Patients taking metronidazole should avoid alcoholic beverages during and for at least 1 day after treatment.

IX. MULTIPLE CHOICE

Circle the letter of the best answer.

1. Which of the following sulfonamides are used to treat second- and third-degree burns?
   a. sulfasoxazole
   b. sulfasalazine
   c. sulfamethoxazole
   d. Sulfamylon
   e. sulfamethizole

2. Sulfonamides can produce which of the following adverse reactions?
   a. crystalluria
   b. hypersensitivity reactions
   c. anorexia
   d. hematological changes
   e. all of the answers are correct

3. The most frequent adverse reaction seen with mafenide is _____ .
   a. stomatitis
   b. burning sensation or pain
   c. fever
   d. increased appetite
   e. lesions on the skin at the injection site

4. The bacteriostatic activity of sulfonamides is due to the sulfonamides' _____ .
   a. activity against the cell wall
   b. activity which inhibits metabolism
   c. overstimulation of cell growth
   d. antagonism to para-aminobenzoic acid
   e. answers a and c are correct

5. When a sulfonamide is given with chlorprop-amide, the sulfonamide may _____ .

   a. decrease the use of glucose
   b. increase the possibility of a hypoglycemic re-action
   c. lose its bacteriostatic ability
   d. increase its effectiveness
   e. none of the answers are correct

6. Sulfonamides are generally administered _____ .

   a. on an empty stomach
   b. with a full glass of water
   c. with acidic fruit juices
   d. with milk or milk products
   e. answers a and b are correct

7. Amoxicillin is an example of a(n) _____ peni-cillin.

   a. natural
   b. penicillinase-resistant
   c. amino-penicillin
   d. extended-spectrum
   e. none of the answers are correct

8. Examples of beta-lactamase inhibitors are all of the following except _____ .

   a. tazobactam
   b. clavulanic acid
   c. ticarcillin
   d. sulbactam
   e. all of the answers are beta-lactamase inhibi-tors

9. Penicillins may be effective against which of the following types of bacteria?

   a. gonococci
   b. staphylococci
   c. streptococci
   d. pneumococci
   e. all of the answers are correct

10. Pseudomembranous colitis is _____ .

    a. a common type of fungal superinfection
    b. a common type of bacterial superinfection
    c. a common type of viral superinfection
    d. caused by an overgrowth of *Clostridium diffi-cile*
    e. answers b and d are correct

11. Intramuscular penicillin injections can cause anaphylactic reactions which are most likely to occur _____ .

    a. in 4–6 days
    b. within 30 minutes
    c. in 4–6 weeks

    d. only after multiple injections
    e. none of the answers are correct

12. Patients experiencing a dermatological reaction as the result of use of penicillin may _____ .

    a. need to continue using the drug if the reac-tion is mild
    b. be prescribed an antihistamine
    c. need to use an antipyretic cream
    d. need to report this reaction to the healthcare provider
    e. all of the answers are correct

13. A first-generation cephalosporin would be more useful against _____ .

    a. Gram-negative organisms
    b. Gram-positive organisms
    c. both Gram-negative and Gram-positive or-ganisms
    d. fungal infections
    e. viral infections only

14. The most common adverse reaction of cephalo-sporins is _____ .

    a. gastrointestinal disturbances
    b. visual disturbances
    c. diabetes
    d. sore throat
    e. ototoxicity

15. Patients receiving cephalosporin therapy should be closely monitored for _____ .

    a. anemia
    b. nephrotoxicity
    c. signs of bacterial or fungal superinfections
    d. hypersensitivity reactions
    e. all of the answers are correct

16. An elderly patient receiving cephalosporin ther-apy who has existing renal impairment would probably need _____ .

    a. a higher dosage of drug and regular liver profile tests
    b. the same dosage of drug as a healthy pa-tient and blood glucose monitoring
    c. a lower dosage of the drug and blood creati-nine level monitoring
    d. a higher dosage of the drug and blood glu-cose monitoring
    e. a lower dosage of the drug and regular liver profile tests

17. Which of the following is not an example of a tetracycline?

    a. Vibramycin
    b. tetracycline

c. doxycycline
d. clarithromycin
e. minocycline

18. Which of the following is an example of a macrolide?
    a. erythromycin
    b. lincomycin
    c. clindamycin
    d. doxycycline
    e. Sumycin

19. Clindamycin is an example of a(n) _____ .
    a. tetracycline
    b. macrolide
    c. cephalosporin
    d. penicillin
    e. lincosamide

20. Tetracyclines are used to treat _____ .
    a. Gram-negative and Gram-positive microorganisms
    b. Rickettsial infections
    c. intestinal amebiasis
    d. uncomplicated *Chlamydia trachomatis* infections
    e. all of the answers are correct

21. Tetracyclines are not given to children younger than 9 years of age unless absolutely necessary because _____ .
    a. it retards their growth
    b. it may cause permanent yellow-gray-brown discoloration of their teeth
    c. it is too nephrotoxic for children
    d. it causes severe gastrointestinal upset
    e. of Stevens-Johnson syndrome

22. Macrolides act by _____ .
    a. binding to cell membranes
    b. causing changes in protein function
    c. inhibiting bacterial replication
    d. answers a and b are correct
    e. answers b and c are correct

23. Macrolides should not be taken with _____ .
    a. clindamycin
    b. lincomycin
    c. chloramphenicol
    d. none of the answers are correct
    e. all of the answers (a–c) are correct

24. Lincosamides are contraindicated in patients with _____ .
    a. hypersensitivity
    b. minor bacterial infections

c. minor viral infections
d. infancy and lactation
e. all of the answers are correct

25. When used with neuromuscular blocking drugs, lincosamides can enhance their effect and possibly lead to _____ .
    a. severe tachycardia
    b. profound respiratory depression
    c. moderate respiratory stimulation
    d. urinary retention
    e. none of the answers are correct

26. Which of the following macrolides should be taken with food or within 1 hour of eating?
    a. erythromycin
    b. dirithromycin
    c. clarithromycin
    d. azithromycin
    e. all of the answers are correct

27. Fluoroquinolones are used to treat _____ infections.
    a. lower respiratory tract
    b. skin
    c. urinary tract
    d. sexually transmitted
    e. all of the answers are correct

28. _____ is an oral aminoglycoside used preoperatively to suppress gastrointestinal bacteria.
    a. Kantrex
    b. Garamycin
    c. Mycifradin
    d. answers a and c are correct
    e. all of the answers (a–c) are correct

29. _____ is used orally in the management of hepatic coma.
    a. Amikacin
    b. Paromomycin
    c. Gentamicin
    d. Tobramycin
    e. Streptomycin

30. _____ produced by aminoglycoside therapy is (are) most often permanent.
    a. Liver damage
    b. Nephrotoxicity
    c. Visual disturbances
    d. Ototoxicity
    e. Answers a and c are correct

31. Mrs. P has been taking an aminoglycoside and reports that her fingers are tingling. This may be indicative of _____ .
    a. respiratory difficulties
    b. neurotoxicity
    c. nephrotoxicity
    d. hypersensitivity reactions
    e. none of the answers are correct

32. Auditory changes in patients taking an aminoglycoside may be _____ .
    a. bilateral
    b. irreversible
    c. partial
    d. total
    e. all of the answers are correct

33. _____ is the only aminoglycoside that cannot be given either intravenously or intramuscularly.
    a. Paromomycin
    b. Streptomycin
    c. Kanamycin
    d. Neomycin
    e. None of the answers are correct

34. Patient education about fluoroquinolone or aminoglycoside therapy is important because it _____ .
    a. encourages compliance
    b. relieves anxiety
    c. promotes the desired result
    d. answers a and c are correct
    e. all of the answers (a–c) are correct

35. Second-line antitubercular drugs are _____ .
    a. less effective than primary drugs
    b. more toxic than primary drugs
    c. used to treat extrapulmonary tuberculosis
    d. used to treat drug-resistant tuberculosis
    e. all of the answers are correct

36. Isoniazid's primary use is _____ .
    a. part of second-line therapy
    b. preventive therapy against tuberculosis
    c. part of primary drug therapy
    d. for treatment of children with tuberculosis
    e. for treating pregnant women with tuberculosis

37. Re-treatment regimens for tuberculosis therapy include all the following drugs except _____ .
    a. capreomycin
    b. cycloserine
    c. isoniazid

    d. aminosalicylic acid
    e. ethionamide

38. Patients taking isoniazid should _____ .
    a. not eat foods with tyramine
    b. not consume alcohol
    c. not use products with aluminum salts
    d. have liver enzyme test
    e. all of the answers are correct

39. _____ is the principal adverse reaction of pyrazinamide use.
    a. Optic neuritis
    b. Hepatotoxicity
    c. Kidney failure
    d. Hypertension
    e. Asthma

40. Streptomycin may cause _____ .
    a. permanent hearing loss
    b. fetal harm
    c. hepatotoxicity
    d. answers a and b are correct
    e. answers b and c are correct

41. Which of the following antitubercular drugs is given daily as an intramuscular injection?
    a. isoniazid
    b. rifampin
    c. streptomycin
    d. ethambutol
    e. pyrazinamide

42. Which of the following antitubercular drugs may cause the patient's urine, feces, or saliva to turn reddish-orange?
    a. ethambutol
    b. isoniazid
    c. rifampin
    d. answers a and c are correct
    e. none of the answers are correct

43. Dapsone is used to treat _____ .
    a. dermatitis
    b. leprosy
    c. tuberculosis
    d. all of the answers (a–c) are correct
    e. answers a and b are correct

44. Chloramphenicol works by _____ .
    a. interfering with or inhibiting protein synthesis
    b. causing cell wall lysis
    c. overstimulating cell growth causing death of the microorganism

d. depleting cellular glycogen stores
e. none of the answers are correct

45. Meropenem is used to treat _____ .
    a. intra-abdominal infections
    b. bacterial meningitis
    c. pseudomembranous colitis
    d. oculitis
    e. answers a and b are correct

46. The most serious adverse reactions of metronidazole involve the _____ .
    a. gastrointestinal tract
    b. central nervous system
    c. ears
    d. kidneys
    e. liver

47. Pentamidine isethionate is used in the treatment of _____ .
    a. *Enterobacter citre*
    b. *Pseudomonas aeruginosa*
    c. *Pneumocystis carinii*
    d. methicillin-resistant *Staphylococcus aureus* (MRSA)
    e. amebiasis

48. Which miscellaneous anti-infective is only given by the intravenous route?
    a. chloramphenicol
    b. meropenem
    c. linezolid
    d. metronidazole
    e. pentamidine isethionate

49. _____ may be given by aerosol.
    a. Chloramphenicol
    b. Meropenem
    c. Linezolid
    d. Metronidazole
    e. Pentamidine isethionate

50. Patients with gynecologic infections, such as trichomoniasis, may be treated with _____ .
    a. chloramphenicol
    b. meropenem
    c. linezolid
    d. metronidazole
    e. pentamidine isethionate

X. RECALL FACTS

Indicate which of the following statements are Facts with an F. If the statement is not a fact, leave the line blank.

About Pseudomembranous Colitis

_____ 1. Is a common bacterial superinfection.

_____ 2. Is a potentially life-threatening problem.

_____ 3. Can also cause candidiasis.

_____ 4. Only occurs with extended drug use.

_____ 5. Is caused by an overgrowth of C. *difficile.*

_____ 6. Is easy to treat.

_____ 7. Has symptoms like diarrhea with blood and mucus.

_____ 8. Usually requires immediate discontinuation of the antibiotic.

_____ 9. May occur 4–9 days after treatment with penicillin.

_____ 10. May occur as long as 6 weeks after discontinuing the drug.

About Cephalosporins

_____ 1. Are classified as Pregnancy Category B drugs.

_____ 2. When taken with oral anticoagulants the risk of bleeding decreases.

_____ 3. Is safe to use alcohol during therapy.

_____ 4. When taken with aminoglycosides the risk of nephrotoxicity increases.

_____ 5. When alcohol is consumed a disulfiram-like reaction may occur.

_____ 6. Should be taken around the clock to maintain blood levels.

_____ 7. May be taken with food.

_____ 8. Examples are cefdinir, cefuroxime, and cefpodoxime.

About Tetracycline Interactions

_____ 1. Counteract the action of aminoglycosides.

_____ 2. May decrease the effect of oral contraceptives.

_____ 3. May increase the effect of oral anticoagulants.

_____ 4. May increase the risk of digitalis toxicity.

_____ 5. Increase the effectiveness of cephalosporins.

_____ 6. May reduce insulin requirements.

About Fluoroquinolone Interactions

_____ 1. Can increase the effects of oral anticoagulants.

_____ 2. Can increase serum theophylline levels.

_____ 3. Can increase cimetidine levels.

_____ 4. Antacids, iron salts, or zinc will increase absorption of fluoroquinolones.

_____ 5. May increase risk of seizure with nonsteroidal anti-inflammatory drugs.

_____ 6. Increased risk of severe cardiac arrhythmias when given with procainamide.

XI. FILL IN THE BLANK

Fill in the blanks using words from the list below.

bacteriostatic	decrease
sulfonamides	alcoholic beverages
beta-lactamase	optic neuritis
stop	increase
silver sulfadiazine	acute gout
cephalosporins	urine output
penicillinase	bacteriocidal
parenteral	myasthenia gravis
ampicillin	fluoroquinolone
minocycline	4
cephalosporins	oral
bacteriostatic	dapsone
impair	liver disease
hour	DNA
nephrotoxicity	pyrazinamide
blood dyscrasias	meropenem
linezolid	vancomycin
gonorrhea	positive

1. Sulfonamides are primarily
   _____ .

2. _____ may produce hematological changes such as agranulocytosis, thrombocytopenia, aplastic anemia, or leukopenia.

3. Any sign of leukopenia or thrombocytopenia in patients taking sulfonamides should be re-

ported immediately because this is an indication to _____ drug therapy.

4. Patients with burns being treated with _____ should have the area inspected every 1–2 hours.

5. _____ is an enzyme produced by certain bacteria that inactivates penicillin.

6. The enzyme _____ is produced by certain bacteria and is able to destroy a component of penicillin.

7. Anaphylactic shock occurs more frequently after _____ use but can occur with _____ use.

8. _____ may interfere with the effectiveness of birth control pills that contain estrogen.

9. _____ are structurally and chemically related to penicillin.

10. The progression from first- to third-generation cephalosporin shows a(n) _____ in sensitivity to Gram-negative organisms and a(n) _____ in sensitivity to Gram-positive organisms.

11. An early sign of nephrotoxicity caused by the use of cephalosporins may be a decreased _____ .

12. Patients receiving cephalosporins should be monitored every _____ hours for fever and impaired skin integrity.

13. In patients who have a history of allergies to penicillins, the _____ are contraindicated.

14. Macrolides and lincosamides may be _____ or _____ .

15. _____ is the tetracycline least likely to cause a photosensitivity reaction.

16. Antacids containing aluminum, zinc, magnesium, or bismuth salts or foods high in calcium _____ absorption of tetracyclines.

17. Macrolides are contraindicated in patients with pre-existing _____ .

18. The neuromuscular blocking action of lincosamides poses a danger to patients with _____ .

19. A patient with an elevated temperature who is taking a tetracycline, macrolide, or lincosamide should be monitored every _____ until the temperature returns to normal.

20. Fluoroquinolones act by interfering with an enzyme needed by the bacteria for _____ synthesis.

21. _____ therapy can cause rupture of the Achilles tendon.

22. A patient taking an aminoglycoside with a urinary output of less than 750 mL/day may be at risk for _____ .

23. A patient receiving aminoglycoside or fluoroquinolone therapy should be cautioned against the use of _____ during therapy.

24. The CDC treatment recommendations for tuberculosis in areas of low incidence for the initial phase includes the use of rifampin, isoniazid, and _____ for a minimum of 2 months.

25. _____ is an adverse reaction of ethambutol which appears to be related to the dose given and the duration of treatment.

26. Pyrazinamide is contraindicated in patients with _____ and severe liver damage.

27. _____ and clofazimine can be used to treat leprosy.

28. The chief adverse reaction seen with the use of chloramphenicol are _____ .

29. _____ is contraindicated in patients with phenylketonuria (PKU).

30. _____ can cause an abscess or phlebitis at the injection site.

31. Spectinomycin is used to treat _____ .

32. Vancomycin acts against susceptible Gram-_____ bacteria.

33. "Red neck" syndrome refers to a severe adverse reaction associated with intravenous use of _____ .

XII. LIST

List the requested number of items.

1. List three bacteria that cause urinary tract infections that sulfonamides are often used to control.
   a. _____
   b. _____
   c. _____

2. List five signs of Stevens-Johnson syndrome.
   a. _____
   b. _____
   c. _____
   d. _____
   e. _____

3. List the four groups of penicillins.
   a. _____
   b. _____

c. _____

d. _____

4. List five types of infections that penicillins may be used to treat.

    a. _____

    b. _____

    c. _____

    d. _____

    e. _____

5. List five adverse reactions of penicillins.

    a. _____

    b. _____

    c. _____

    d. _____

    e. _____

6. List six infectious organisms that cephalosporins may be used to treat.

    a. _____

    b. _____

    c. _____

    d. _____

    e. _____

    f. _____

7. List five adverse reactions of lincosamides.

    a. _____

    b. _____

    c. _____

    d. _____

    e. _____

8. List five products that should not be taken with tetracyclines.

    a. _____

    b. _____

    c. _____

    d. _____

    e. _____

9. List five examples of fluoroquinolones.

    a. _____

    b. _____

    c. _____

    d. _____

    e. _____

10. List five potential adverse reactions of aminoglycosides.

    a. _____

    b. _____

    c. _____

    d. _____

    e. _____

11. List five aminoglycosides that are Pregnancy Category D drugs.

    a. _____

    b. _____

    c. _____

    d. _____

    e. _____

12. List three fluoroquinolones that may be given intravenously.

    a. _____

    b. _____

    c. _____

13. List five drugs that can be used in the initial phase of standard treatment for tuberculosis.

    a. _____

    b. _____

    c. _____

    d. _____

    e. _____

14. List four uses of linezolid.

    a. _____

    b. _____

    c. _____

    d. _____

15. List seven miscellaneous anti-infectives.

a. _____

b. _____

c. _____

d. _____

e. _____

f. _____

g. _____

16. List six microorganisms that meropenem can be used to treat.

a. _____

b. _____

c. _____

d. _____

e. _____

f. _____

XIII. CLINICAL APPLICATIONS

1. Miss P, age 83, cannot remember if she is allergic to penicillin. What symptoms might you ask her about to help determine if she has had a hypersensitivity reaction to these drugs in the past?

2. Mrs. R has been prescribed a cephalosporin for her infection. She has been advised to be on the alert for a superinfection but does not know what the symptoms of this are. Explain to Mrs. R and her family what she should look for.

26 Other Anti-Infective Drugs

I. MATCHING

Match the term from Column A with the correct definition from Column B.

COLUMN A

_____ 1. anthelmintic

_____ 2. cinchonism

_____ 3. fungicidal

_____ 4. helminthiasis

_____ 5. mycotic infection

_____ 6. onychomycosis

_____ 7. parasite

_____ 8. tinea corporis

COLUMN B

A. A group of symptoms associated with quinine.
B. Invasion of the body by helminths.
C. Jock itch.
D. Drugs with actions against helminths.
E. A superficial or deep infection caused by a fungi disease in humans that may be yeastlike or moldlike.
F. Able to destroy fungi.
G. Nail fungus condition.
H. An organism that lives in or on another organism without contributing to the survival or well-being of the host.

II. MATCHING

Match the generic antiviral drug in Column A with the correct trade name in Column B.

COLUMN A

_____ 1. acyclovir

_____ 2. cidofovir

_____ 3. valganciclovir

_____ 4. imiquimod

_____ 5. zanamivir

_____ 6. didanosine

_____ 7. lopinavir/ritonavir

_____ 8. oseltamivir

_____ 9. zidovudine (AZT)

_____ 10. famciclovir

_____ 11. amantadine

_____ 12. ritonavir

_____ 13. stavudine

_____ 14. vidarabine

_____ 15. docosanol

COLUMN B

A. Videx
B. Tamiflu
C. Aldara
D. Norvir
E. Retrovir
F. Abreva
G. Valcyte
H. Symmetrel
I. Zovirax
J. Kaletra
K. Ara-A, Vira-A
L. Famvir
M. Zerit
N. Relenza
O. Vistide

III. MATCHING

Match the generic antifungal drug in Column A with the correct trade name in Column B.

COLUMN A

_____ 1. itraconazole

_____ 2. ketoconazole

_____ 3. fluconazole

_____ 4. amphotericin B desoxycholate

_____ 5. flucytosine (5-FC)

_____ 6. caspofungin acetate

_____ 7. griseofulvin microsize

_____ 8. amphotericin B, lipid-based

COLUMN B

A. Diflucan
B. Ancobon
C. Nizoral
D. Sporanox
E. Grisactin
F. Cancidas
G. Amphocin
H. Abelcet

IV. MATCHING

Match the generic topical antifungal drug in Column A with the correct trade name in Column B.

COLUMN A

_____ 1. naftifine

_____ 2. undecylenic acid

_____ 3. miconazole nitrate (cream)

_____ 4. clotrimazole

_____ 5. haloprogin

_____ 6. tolnaftate

_____ 7. butenafine HCl

_____ 8. amphotericin B (cream)

COLUMN B

A. Lotrimin
B. Fungizone
C. Mentax
D. Aftate
E. Naftin
F. Cruex
G. Halotex
H. Monistat

V. MATCHING

Match the generic anthelmintic, antimalarial, or amebicide in Column A with the correct trade name in Column B.

COLUMN A

_____ 1. halofantrine

_____ 2. metronidazole

_____ 3. atovaquone and proguanil HCl

_____ 4. pyrimethamine

_____ 5. mebendazole

_____ 6. sulfadoxine and pyrimethamine

_____ 7. mefloquine hydrochloride

_____ 8. thiabendazole

_____ 9. paromomycin

_____ 10. chloroquine hydrochloride

_____ 11. iodoquinol

_____ 12. pyrantel

COLUMN B

A. Daraprim
B. Flagyl
C. Mintezol
D. Aralen
E. Lariam
F. Malarone
G. Vermox
H. Humatin
I. Halfan
J. Fansidar
K. Yodoxin
L. Reese's pinworm

VI. MATCHING

Match the trade name in Column A with the type of anti-infective in Column B. You may use an answer more than once.

COLUMN A

_____ 1. Denavir

_____ 2. AmBisome

_____ 3. Antiminth

_____ 4. Agenerase

_____ 5. Nizoral

_____ 6. Halotex

_____ 7. Exelderm

_____ 8. Mintezol

_____ 9. Desenex

_____ 10. Monodox

_____ 11. Rescriptor

_____ 12. Foscavir

_____ 13. Femstat 3

_____ 14. Lotrimin 3

_____ 15. Fansidar

_____ 16. Aralen

_____ 17. Yodoxin

COLUMN B

A. Antiviral
B. Antifungal
C. Topical antifungal
D. Vaginal antifungal
E. Anthelmintic
F. Antimalarial
G. Amebicide

VII. MATCHING

Match the antiviral trade name in Column A with the correct use in Column B. You may use an answer more than once.

COLUMN A

_____ 1. Valcyte

_____ 2. Cytovene

_____ 3. Famvir

_____ 4. Ara-A

_____ 5. Virazole

_____ 6. Aldara

_____ 7. Relenza

_____ 8. Abreva

_____ 9. Ziagen

_____ 10. Denavir

_____ 11. Sustiva

_____ 12. Videx

_____ 13. Flumadine

_____ 14. Zerit

COLUMN B

A. Acute herpes zoster
B. Severe lower respiratory tract infection
C. Influenza virus
D. Keratitis
E. HSV types 1 and 2
F. CMV retinitis
G. HIV
H. Influenza A virus
I. External genitalia and perianal warts

VIII. MATCHING

Match the trade name of the anthelmintic, antimalarial, or amebicide drug in Column A with the correct use in Column B. You may use an answer more than once.

COLUMN A

_____ 1. Flagyl

_____ 2. Vibra-Tabs

_____ 3. Albenza

_____ 4. Vermox

_____ 5. Humatin

_____ 6. Plaquenil sulfate

_____ 7. Mintezol

_____ 8. quinine sulfate

_____ 9. Antiminth

COLUMN B

A. Treatment of threadworm
B. Treatment of intestinal amebiasis
C. Treatment of malaria
D. Prevention and treatment of malaria
E. Short-term prevention of malaria
F. American hookworm, whipworm, pinworm, roundworm
G. Hydatid disease
H. Roundworm and pinworm

IX. MATCHING

Match the fungicide in Column A with the mode of action in Column B. You may use an answer more than once or not at all.

COLUMN A

_____ 1. Diflucan

_____ 2. Lotrimin

_____ 3. Grisactin

_____ 4. Nizoral

_____ 5. Monistat

_____ 6. Ancobon

_____ 7. Fungizone IV

_____ 8. Mycostatin

_____ 9. Mycelex

COLUMN B

A. Not clearly understood
B. Is deposited in keratin precursor cells which are then lost and replaced by uninfected cells
C. Effect on cell membrane
D. Causes depletion of sterols
E. Related to concentration in body tissues
F. Causes cells to die
G. Binds with phospholipids in fungal cell membrane increasing permeability of the cell

X. MATCHING

Match the anthelmintic drug in Column A with the action in Column B.

COLUMN A

_____ 1. albendazole

_____ 2. mebendazole

_____ 3. pyrantel

_____ 4. thiabendazole

COLUMN B

A. Interferes with the synthesis of the parasites microtubules
B. Blocks the uptake of glucose by the helminth
C. Appears to suppress egg or larval production
D. Paralyzes the helminth

XI. TRUE/FALSE

Indicate whether each statement is True (T) or False (F).

_____ 1. Most antiviral drugs act by inhibiting viral DNA or RNA replication in the virus.

_____ 2. All antiviral drugs are contraindicated in patients with congestive heart failure and during lactation.

_____ 3. A rash at the site of application is a normal reaction to a topical antiviral drug.

_____ 4. Acyclovir, in any form of administration, has no precautions; it is safe for everyone to use.

_____ 5. Symptoms of pancreatitis or peripheral neuropathy that appear during the use of didanosine should be reported immediately to the healthcare provider.

_____ 6. Didanosine tablets should be chewed or crushed and mixed with water.

_____ 7. Zanamivir can cause serious adverse reactions such as bronchospasm, which can lead to death.

_____ 8. A mycotic infection is caused by a plant that contains chlorophyll.

_____ 9. Deep mycotic infections are among the easiest to treat because of their limited location.

_____ 10. Topical antifungal drugs generally cause few adverse reactions.

_____ 11. Some adverse reactions of amphotericin B may be lessened by the use of aspirin, antihistamines, or antiemetics.

_____ 12. Amphotericin B may be nephrotoxic.

_____ 13. Fluconazole can alter liver function.

_____ 14. Gastrointestinal distress is rarely a problem with flucytosine use.

_____ 15. Griseofulvin may produce a rash and urticaria as part of a hypersensitivity reaction.

_____ 16. Patients may develop hepatitis during itraconazole use.

_____ 17. Few patients can tolerate ketoconazole without severe adverse reactions.

_____ 18. Tea tree oil is an effective antifungal that is used to relieve and control the symptoms of tinea pedis.

_____ 19. Albenza works by interfering with the synthesis of the parasite's microtubules.

_____ 20. The four anthelmintic drugs discussed in Chapter 26 are all Pregnancy Category B drugs.

_____ 21. Mebendazole can cause leukopenia or thrombocytopenia.

_____ 22. Diarrhea is a common adverse reaction of anthelmintic drugs.

_____ 23. Malaria is caused by the protozoan species *Anopheles*.

_____ 24. The symptoms of malaria appear when the sporozoites enter the person's bloodstream.

_____ 25. Aralen is only used in the treatment of malaria.

_____ 26. All antimalarial drugs work equally well in suppressing or treating all four of the *Plasmodium* species that cause malaria.

_____ 27. Chloroquine should be used with extreme caution in children.

_____ 28. Doxycycline is a Pregnancy Category D drug.

_____ 29. Quinine is contraindicated in pregnant women and in patients with myasthenia gravis.

_____ 30. Visual disturbances observed in patients taking chloroquine have caused no long-term problems.

_____ 31. Amebicides kill amebas.

_____ 32. Extraintestinal amebiasis is more difficult to treat.

_____ 33. Metronidazole can cause convulsive seizures and peripheral neuropathy.

_____ 34. Rare but serious adverse reactions of paromomycin are nephrotoxicity and ototoxicity.

_____ 35. It is common practice to test immediate family members for amebiasis.

XII. MULTIPLE CHOICE

Circle the letter of the best answer.

1. Antiviral drugs may be given as _____ .
   a. topical drugs
   b. systemic drugs
   c. oral drugs
   d. intravenous drugs
   e. all of the answers are correct

2. The most common adverse reaction(s) of antiviral drugs that are administered systemically are _____ .
   a. visual disturbances
   b. gastrointestinal disturbances
   c. reproductive difficulties
   d. CNS depression
   e. musculoskeletal twitching

3. The antiviral drug _____ is a Pregnancy Category X drug.
   a. ribavirin
   b. amprenavir
   c. ganciclovir
   d. imiquimod
   e. ritonavir

4. Acyclovir _____ .
   a. can be used orally, topically, or parenterally
   b. can cause crystalluria if adequate hydration is not maintained
   c. treatment should begin as soon as symptoms of herpes simplex appear
   d. can be given without regard to food
   e. all of the answers are correct

5. Amantadine is used with caution in all of the following conditions except _____ .
   a. seizure disorders
   b. psychiatric problems
   c. emphysema
   d. kidney impairment
   e. cardiac disease

6. Amantadine patients should be monitored for which of the following?
   a. mood changes
   b. thrombocytopenia
   c. liver function
   d. cardiac output
   e. polycythemia

7. Amantadine is used _____ .
   a. to treat HIV
   b. for herpes simplex viral infections
   c. to manage the extrapyramidal effects of drugs used to treat Parkinsonism
   d. for the prevention and treatment of respiratory tract illness caused by influenza type A virus
   e. answers c and d are correct

8. Ribavirin _____ .
   a. is a Pregnancy Category X drug
   b. can cause worsening of respiratory status
   c. is safe to use in patients with COPD
   d. can antagonize the action of zidovudine
   e. all of the answers, except c, are correct

9. Zidovudine _____ .
   a. levels are decreased when given with clarithromycin
   b. levels are increased when give with lamivudine
   c. decreases the neurotoxic effects of acyclovir
   d. answers a and b are correct
   e. answers b and c are correct

10. Lemon balm (*Melissa officinalis*) traditionally has been used _____ .
    a. for Grave's disease
    b. as a sedative

c. as an antispasmodic
d. as an antiviral agent
e. all of the answers are correct

11. Fungal infections may be _____ .

    a. superficial
    b. systemic
    c. intradermal
    d. answers a and b are correct
    e. answers b and c are correct

12. All of the following are examples of superficial mycotic infections except one. Identify the exception.

    a. hydatid disease
    b. onychomycosis
    c. tinea cruris
    d. tinea pedis
    e. tinea corporis

13. Amphotericin B _____ .

    a. is given parenterally
    b. is given for several months
    c. use often results in serious reactions
    d. is reserved for serious and potentially life-threatening fungal infections
    e. all of the answers are correct

14. All of the following statements about amphotericin B are true except one. Identify the exception.

    a. Amphotericin B is given only under close supervision in the hospital.
    b. Amphotericin B can cause severe bone marrow depression.
    c. When given with corticosteroids, amphotericin B may cause hyperkalemia.
    d. Amphotericin B is a Pregnancy Category B drug and is used cautiously during lactation.
    e. Amphotericin B is used cautiously in patients with renal dysfunction or electrolyte imbalances.

15. Fluconazole _____ .

    a. may decrease the metabolism of phenytoin and warfarin
    b. may cause an increased effect of an oral hypoglycemic
    c. may be given orally or intravenously
    d. is considered to be a Pregnancy Category B drug
    e. all of the answers, except d, are correct

16. Flucytosine may have _____ as an adverse reaction.

    a. anemia
    b. leucopenia
    c. thrombocytopenia
    d. answers a and c are correct
    e. all of the answers are correct

17. A patient taking griseofulvin may have a decreased effect of the drug when which of the following drugs are taken concurrently?

    a. warfarin
    b. barbiturate
    c. oral contraceptives
    d. salicylate concentrations
    e. all of the answers are correct

18. Itraconazole _____ .

    a. can be given orally with food to increase absorption
    b. can be used topically
    c. is often diluted with saline for intravenous infusion
    d. should be given with milk
    e. is often given on an empty stomach to increase absorption

19. Ketoconazole _____ .

    a. is commonly given with food
    b. is commonly given with antacids, anticholinergics, or histamine blockers
    c. usually causes severe adverse reactions
    d. is a Pregnancy Category B drug
    e. all of the answers are correct

20. Miconazole _____ .

    a. is used to treat vulvovaginal fungal infections
    b. is used during the first trimester only when essential
    c. may cause irritation, sensitization, or vulvovaginal burning
    d. is usually self-administered on an outpatient basis
    e. all of the answers are correct

21. Which of the following herbs have been identified as being effective against tinea pedis?

    a. oral ingestion of garlic tablets
    b. 10% tea tree oil cream
    c. 0.4% ajoene cream
    d. answers b and c are correct
    e. all of the answers are correct

22. All the following drugs are considered to be anthelmintic drugs except _____ .

    a. albendazole
    b. itraconazole

c. mebendazole
d. pyrantel
e. thiabendazole

23. Which of the following anthelmintic drugs have been shown to cause embryotoxic and teratogenic effects in experimental animals?

   a. albendazole and pyrantel
   b. mebendazole and thiabendazole
   c. albendazole and mebendazole
   d. pyrantel and thiabendazole
   e. mebendazole and pyrantel

24. Which anthelmintic drug may be taken without regard to food?

   a. mebendazole
   b. thiabendazole
   c. albendazole
   d. pyrantel
   e. all of the drugs should be taken with food to increase absorption

25. Doxycycline _____ .

   a. is contraindicated during pregnancy
   b. absorption is decreased when taken with antacids or iron
   c. is an antibiotic
   d. is used to treat malaria
   e. all of the answers are correct

26. When chloroquine is used for prophylaxis, therapy should begin _____ weeks before exposure and continue for _____ weeks after exposure.

   a. 2, 6–8
   b. 4, 1–2
   c. 6, 2
   d. 6–8, 2
   e. 10, 10

27. A patient taking chloroquine may experience which of the following visual disturbances?

   a. disturbed color vision
   b. blurred vision
   c. night blindness
   d. diminished visual fields
   e. all of the answers are correct

28. Which of the following drugs are used to treat intestinal amebiasis?

   a. Aralen
   b. Miconazole
   c. Doxycycline
   d. Yodoxin
   e. pyrantel

29. All of the following drugs are used to treat amebiasis except _____ .

   a. iodoquinol
   b. Vibramycin
   c. metronidazole
   d. paromomycin
   e. chloroquine hydrochloride

30. Patients taking amebicides _____ .

   a. may be at risk for dehydration
   b. may need to have their body weight checked daily
   c. may prefer more frequent smaller meals
   d. may need to have stool specimens saved for laboratory analysis
   e. all of the answers are correct

XIII. RECALL FACTS

Indicate which of the following statements are Facts with an F. If the statement is not a fact, leave the line blank.

About Educating the Patient and Family About Antiviral Drugs

_____ 1. These drugs cure viral infections.

_____ 2. These drugs should decrease the symptoms of viral infections.

_____ 3. A missed dose should not be doubled at the next dosage time.

_____ 4. Symptoms of infection should be reported.

_____ 5. It is common practice to stop the medication once the patient feels better.

_____ 6. Signs of pancreatitis need to be reported immediately.

_____ 7. Peripheral neuropathy is to be expected and tolerated by the patient.

About General Patient Management Issues with Antifungal Drugs

_____ 1. Oral and parenteral drug routes require patient observation every 2–4 hours for adverse reactions.

_____ 2. Topical antifungal drug use should be monitored weekly.

_____ 3. Antifungal drug therapy may require weeks to months.

_____ 4. Drugs that are potentially toxic to the kidneys only require fluid monitoring.

_____ 5. Serum creatinine and blood urea nitrogen levels should be checked frequently during therapy.

_____ 6. Gloves should be used when caring for open lesions.

XIV. FILL IN THE BLANK

Fill in the blanks using words from the list below.

zidovudine	*Candida albicans*
inhalation	fungus
topical	unlabeled
decreased	2
amphotericin B	kidney damage
diabetes	reduce
oral thrush	fluconazole
anthelmintic drugs	hepatotoxicity
flucytosine	exactly
intestinal	delayed
cinchonism	acidify
antimalarial	pyrantel
Flagyl	iodoquinol
alcohol	bowel
amebiasis	X

1. The use of a drug for a specific disorder or condition that is not officially approved by the FDA is called a(n) _____ use.

2. _____ administration of antiviral drugs can cause transient burning, stinging, and pruritus as adverse reactions.

3. Absorption of didanosine is _____ when it is administered with food.

4. Ribavirin is given by _____ .

5. Zanamivir drug therapy should be started within _____ days' onset of flu symptoms.

6. _____ drug therapy can cause hematological changes such as anemia, granulocytopenia, and bone marrow depression.

7. A(n) _____ is a colorless plant that lacks chlorophyll.

8. _____ commonly causes yeast infections in women.

9. _____ is the most effective drug available for the treatment of most systemic fungal infections.

10. _____ is the most serious adverse reaction of amphotericin B.

11. _____ may increase an older patient's risk of decreased renal and liver function.

12. Before therapy is begun with _____, the patient's hematological, electrolyte, and renal status are determined.

13. Griseofulvin can cause _____ to occur.

14. Itraconazole and ketoconazole use may cause _____ .

15. Patients with recurrent or chronic cases of candidiasis who repeatedly are prescribed miconazole should be evaluated for _____ .

16. The prime purpose of _____ is to kill the parasite.

17. Use of mebendazole with the hydantoins and carbamazepine may _____ plasma levels of mebendazole.

18. _____ and piperazine are antagonists and should not be given together.

19. _____ drugs interfere with the life cycle of the plasmodium, primarily when it is present in red blood cells.

20. Foods that _____ the urine may increase excretion and decrease the effectiveness of chloroquine.

21. The use of quinine can cause _____ at full therapeutic doses.

22. Quinine is a Pregnancy Category _____ drug.

23. Quinine absorption is _____ when taken with antacids containing aluminum.

24. Antimalarial drugs taken for suppression of malaria should be taken _____ as prescribed.

25. The two types of amebiasis are _____ and extraintestinal.

26. _____ is used to treat intestinal amebiasis.

27. _____ may interfere with thyroid function tests for as long as 6 months after therapy is discontinued.

28. Patients taking metronidazole must avoid _____ while undergoing treatment.

29. Paromomycin is given with caution to patients with _____ disease.

30. Patients with _____ may or may not be acutely ill and may require isolation procedures.

XV. LIST

List the requested number of items.

1. List seven uses of antiviral drugs.
   a. _____
   b. _____
   c. _____
   d. _____
   e. _____
   f. _____
   g. _____

2. List five drugs that when used concurrently with amantadine may increase its anticholinergic effects.
   a. _____
   b. _____
   c. _____
   d. _____
   e. _____

3. List five examples of helminths.
   a. _____
   b. _____
   c. _____
   d. _____
   e. _____

4. List three precautions that should be taken by the healthcare worker when dealing with a patient who has a helminth infection.
   a. _____
   b. _____
   c. _____

5. List the four protozoans that can cause malaria.
   a. _____
   b. _____
   c. _____
   d. _____

6. List six adverse reactions of chloroquine.
   a. _____
   b. _____
   c. _____
   d. _____
   e. _____
   f. _____

7. List five symptoms of cinchonism.

a. _____

b. _____

c. _____

d. _____

e. _____

8. List five conditions that put women at risk for vulvovaginal yeast infections.

a. _____

b. _____

c. _____

d. _____

e. _____

9. List five adverse reactions of amphotericin B.

a. _____

b. _____

c. _____

d. _____

e. _____

10. List four drugs that interact with itraconazole and cause a decrease in the blood levels of itraconazole.

a. _____

b. _____

c. _____

d. _____

XVI. CLINICAL APPLICATIONS

1. Miss P has been diagnosed with a herpes simplex infection. She is to take the oral medication (Zovirax) for her treatment. Explain to Miss P what precautions she must follow while taking this medication.

2. Mrs. C's daughter, who is 17 years old, has been invited to participate in a school trip to an area that has malaria. The school nurse has sent a note home with the students which states that they must see their family physician soon to get started on the required medication for the trip. Explain to Mrs. C the types of treatments used for malaria and why it is important for her daughter to take the medication exactly as prescribed.

27 Immunological Agents

I. MATCHING

Match the term from Column A with the correct definition from Column B.

COLUMN A

_____ 1. antibody

_____ 2. antigen

_____ 3. attenuated

_____ 4. globulin

_____ 5. toxin

_____ 6. toxoid

_____ 7. vaccine

_____ 8. booster

COLUMN B

A. The administration of an additional dose of the vaccine to "boost" the production of antibodies to a level that will maintain the desired immunity.

B. A poisonous substance produced by some bacteria.

C. A toxin that is weakened but still capable of stimulating the formation of antitoxins.

D. A substance, usually a protein, that stimulates the body to produce antibodies.

E. Proteins present in blood serum or plasma that contain antibodies.

F. A globulin produced by the B lymphocytes as a defense against an antigen.

G. Weakened, as in the antigen strain used for vaccine development.

H. Artificial active immunity created with killed or weakened antigens for the purpose of creating resistance to disease.

II. MATCHING

Match the term from Column A with the correct definition from Column B.

COLUMN A

_____ 1. active immunity

_____ 2. cell-mediated immunity

_____ 3. humoral immunity

_____ 4. immunity

_____ 5. passive immunity

_____ 6. immune globulin

COLUMN B

A. Based on the antigen–antibody response, special lymphocytes produce circulating antibodies to act against a foreign substance.

B. The ability of the body to identify and resist microorganism that are potentially harmful.

C. The reaction of the body, when exposed to certain infectious microorganisms, of forming antibodies to the invading microorganism.

D. Solutions obtained from human blood containing antibodies that have been formed by the body to specific antigen.

E. A type of immunity occurring from the administration of ready-made antibodies from another individual or animal.

F. The process of T lymphocytes and macrophages working together to destroy an antigen.

III. MATCHING

Match the generic bacterial vaccine for active immunity in Column A with the correct trade name in Column B.

COLUMN A

_____ 1. typhoid vaccine

_____ 2. pneumococcal 7-valent conjugate vaccine

_____ 3. *Haemophilus influenza* type b conjugate and hepatitis B vaccine

_____ 4. Lyme disease vaccine

_____ 5. pneumococcal vaccine, polyvalent

_____ 6. BCG vaccine

_____ 7. Meningococcal polysaccharide vaccine

COLUMN B

A. Comvax
B. LYMErix
C. Tice BCG
D. Prevnar

E. Pneumovax 23
F. Typhim Vi
G. Menomune A/C/Y/W-135

IV. MATCHING

Match the generic viral vaccine in Column A with the correct trade name in Column B.

COLUMN A

_____ 1. rubella and mumps virus vaccine, live

_____ 2. rubella virus vaccine, live

_____ 3. poliovirus vaccine, inactivated

_____ 4. hepatitis A, inactivated and hepatitis B recombinant vaccine

_____ 5. poliovirus vaccine, live, trivalent, oral

_____ 6. Japanese encephalitis virus vaccine

_____ 7. rotavirus vaccine

_____ 8. varicella virus vaccine

_____ 9. hepatitis B vaccine, recombinant

_____ 10. hepatitis A vaccine

COLUMN B

A. Orimune
B. Rotashield
C. Meruvax II
D. IPOL
E. JE-VAX
F. Biavax-11
G. Havrix
H. Varivax
I. Twinrix
J. Engerix-B

V. MATCHING

Match the generic immune globulin for passive immunity in Column A with the correct trade name in Column B.

COLUMN A

_____ 1. rabies immune globulin, human

_____ 2. cytomegalovirus immune globulin IV, human

_____ 3. Rh (D) immune globulin IV (human)

_____ 4. gamma globulin

_____ 5. lymphocyte immune globulin, antithymocyte globulin (equine)

_____ 6. tetanus immune globulin

_____ 7. respiratory syncytial virus immune globulin IV

_____ 8. hepatitis B immune globulin (human)

_____ 9. Crotalidae polyvalent immune Fab

COLUMN B

A. BayGam
B. WinRho SDF
C. Bay Rab
D. Atgam
E. RespiGam
F. CytoGam
G. BayTet
H. BayHep B
I. CroFab

VI. MATCHING

Match the trade name in Column A with the type of immunity in Column B. You may use an answer more than once.

COLUMN A

_____ 1. Havrix

_____ 2. Imovax Rabies I.D.

_____ 3. BayGam

_____ 4. Act HIB

_____ 5. Atgam

_____ 6. FluShield

_____ 7. RespiGam

_____ 8. CroFab

_____ 9. Prevnar

_____ 10. Gamulin Rh

_____ 11. Certiva

_____ 12. Mumpsvax

COLUMN B

A. Active
B. Passive

VII. MATCHING

Match the trade name in Column A with the type of agent in Column B. You may use an answer more than once.

COLUMN A

_____ 1. Meruvax II

_____ 2. WinRho SDF

_____ 3. Cholera vaccine

_____ 4. Typhim Vi

_____ 5. M-R-Vax II

_____ 6. Atgam

_____ 7. CroFab

_____ 8. Certiva

_____ 9. TriHIBit

_____ 10. CytoGam

_____ 11. YF-Vax

_____ 12. Bay Tet

_____ 13. Vaqta

_____ 14. Attenuvax

_____ 15. Pediatrix

COLUMN B

A. Bacterial vaccine
B. Viral vaccine
C. Toxoid
D. Immune globulin
E. Antivenin

VIII. TRUE/FALSE

Indicate whether each statement is True (T) or False (F).

_____ 1. Active immunity involves agents that stimulate antibody formation.

_____ 2. Immunity is the resistance that an individual has against disease.

_____ 3. A vaccine that contains an attenuated antigen is one in which the antigen has been killed.

_____ 4. Many antigens, when killed, cause a good antibody response.

_____ 5. All forms of active immunity require booster shots.

_____ 6. Antibody-producing tissues cannot distinguish between a live or dead antigen.

_____ 7. Vaccines that contain weakened antigens are capable of causing disease in healthy individuals.

_____ 8. Vaccinations always result in a protective antibody response.

_____ 9. The administration of immune globulins is an example of passive immunity.

_____ 10. Adverse reactions of vaccines and toxoids are usually mild and subside within 48 hours.

_____ 11. The risk of serious adverse reactions from immunizations is much larger than the risk of contracting the same disease.

_____ 12. Immune globulins stimulate antibody production.

_____ 13. For the most effective response, antivenins should be administered within 4 hours after exposure.

_____ 14. A patient with isolated immunoglobulin A deficiency should not be given immune globulin preparations.

_____ 15. Antivenins are contraindicated in patients with hypersensitivity to horse serum or any component of the serum.

_____ 16. Antivenins have multiple known interactions.

_____ 17. All vaccines can be administered to those with minor illness, including a viral cold or a low-grade fever.

_____ 18. A postponement of the regular immunization schedule for children is never indicated.

_____ 19. After injection of immunizations, it is not uncommon to feel a lump at the injection site.

_____ 20. Only incidents that are positively related to an immunization should be reported to the Vaccine Adverse Event Reporting System (VAERS).

_____ 21. Immunizations required for travel should be given well in advance of departure so that adequate immunity is produced.

_____ 22. Serious viral infections of the CNS and fatalities have occurred with the use of some vaccines.

_____ 23. Lentinan may boost the body's immune system and lower cholesterol.

_____ 24. Echinacea should not be taken for more than 8 consecutive weeks.

IX. MULTIPLE CHOICE

Circle the letter of the best answer.

1. _____ immunity occurs when a person is exposed to a disease, experiences the disease, and the body manufactures antibodies.
   a. Artificially acquired active
   b. Attenuated
   c. Passive
   d. Naturally acquired active
   e. Toxoid

2. Passive immunity _____ .
   a. is obtained from the administration of immune globulins or antivenins
   b. provides immediate immunity
   c. lasts for a short time
   d. provides ready-made antibodies from another human or animal
   e. all of the answers are correct

3. Immunological agents may include _____ .
   a. immune globulins
   b. toxoids
   c. vaccines
   d. answers a and b are correct
   e. all of the answers are correct

4. A toxin is _____ .
   a. capable of stimulating the body to produce antibodies
   b. capable of stimulating the body to produce antitoxins
   c. only able to stimulate the production of toxoids
   d. a way to produce antigens
   e. none of the answers are correct

5. Vaccines and toxoids _____ .
   a. are administered to stimulate the immune response in the body
   b. must be administered before exposure to the pathogenic organism
   c. provide passive immunity
   d. answers a and b are correct
   e. answers a and c are correct

6. Mr. C was given hepatitis B immune globulin 60 days ago after being exposed to the virus. He came into the office today to get a Meruvax II vaccine. What should the healthcare provider tell Mr. C?
   a. It is okay to get this vaccine today.
   b. Come back in another 30 days.
   c. The globulin preparation may interfere with your response to the vaccination.
   d. Answers b and c are correct
   e. Mr. C should never get this vaccine.

7. Insufficient antibodies may be produced when the immune system of a patient is depressed because of all but which of the following causes?
   a. corticosteroids
   b. salicylates
   c. antineoplastic drugs
   d. radiation therapy
   e. answers a and b are correct

8. Immune globulins _____ .
   a. provide passive immunity to one or more infectious diseases
   b. produce a rapid onset of protection
   c. provide protection of short duration
   d. are generally given after exposure to the disease
   e. all of the answers are correct

9. Live virus vaccines should be administered 14–30 days before or _____ .
   a. 6–12 weeks after administration of immunoglobulins
   b. 1–2 days after administration of immunoglobulins
   c. 8–10 months after administration of immunoglobulins
   d. not at all after administration of immunoglobulins
   e. 1–2 years after administration of immunoglobulins

10. After administration of an immunological agent _____ .

    a. a patient must be hospitalized for several days
    b. a patient may immediately go home
    c. a patient may be asked to remain on site for approximately 30 minutes
    d. a patient should eat a heavy fat meal
    e. none of the answers are correct

11. _____ is (are) sometimes prescribed every 4 hours to control minor adverse reactions.

    a. Salicylates
    b. Narcotic agents
    c. Analeptics
    d. Acetaminophen
    e. Sedatives

12. The Vaccine Adverse Event Reporting System is a _____ .

    a. local agency that monitors use of vaccines.
    b. way to report healthcare provider carelessness
    c. national vaccine safety surveillance program
    d. program cosponsored by the CDC and the FDA
    e. answers c and d are correct

13. Echinacea is taken to _____ .

    a. stimulate the immune system
    b. increase the number of immune cells
    c. increase the activity of immune cells
    d. stimulate phagocytosis
    e. all of the answers are correct

X. RECALL FACTS

Indicate which of the following statements are Facts with an F. If the statement is not a fact, leave the line blank.

About Contraindications with the MMR Vaccine

_____ 1. Lactation

_____ 2. First trimester of pregnancy

_____ 3. Allergic to neomycin

_____ 4. Allergic to gelatin

_____ 5. Corticosteroid therapy

_____ 6. Second or third trimester of pregnancy

_____ 7. Allergic reaction to previous dose of one of vaccines

_____ 8. Hypersensitive to agent or components

_____ 9. Salicylate administration

_____ 10. Allergies to animals

About Adverse Reactions of Antivenins

_____ 1. Apprehension

_____ 2. Tingling fingers

_____ 3. Usually occur within 30 minutes of administration

_____ 4. Diarrhea

_____ 5. Cyanosis

_____ 6. Collapse

_____ 7. Clubbed fingers

_____ 8. Flushing

_____ 9. Itching and hives

_____ 10. Edema of face, tongue, and throat

XI. FILL IN THE BLANK

Fill in the blanks using words from the list below.

vaccines	increased
toxin	artificially acquired
passive	active
booster	Echinacea
globulins	lentinan
antivenins	measles
mumps	rubella

1. _____ immunity involves the injection of ready-made antibodies found in the serum of immune individuals or animals.

2. _____ active immunity occurs when an individual is given a killed or weakened antigen that stimulates the formation of antibodies.

3. _____ injections help keep an adequate antibody titer circulating in the body.

4. _____ can contain either an attenuated or killed antigen.

5. A _____ is a poisonous substance produced by some bacteria.

6. _____ immunity can be produced by administering vaccines or toxoids.

7. There is a(n) _____ risk of Reye's syndrome when salicylates are administered with the varicella vaccine.

8. _____ are proteins present in blood serum or plasma that contain antibodies.

9. _____ are used for passive, transient protection from the toxic effects of bites by spiders and snakes.

10. Antibodies in immune globulin preparations may interfere with the immune response to live viral vaccines such as _____, _____, and _____.

11. _____ is a derivative of the shiitake mushroom.

12. Persons with allergies to daisy-type plants are more susceptible to adverse reactions to _____ use.

XII. LIST

List the requested number of items.

1. List eight diseases for which there are vaccines available.

    a. _____

    b. _____

    c. _____

    d. _____

    e. _____

    f. _____

    g. _____

    h. _____

2. List five uses of vaccines and toxoids.

    a. _____

    b. _____

    c. _____

    d. _____

    e. _____

3. List five conditions in which vaccine and toxoid use are contraindicated.

    a. _____

    b. _____

    c. _____

    d. _____

    e. _____

4. List five types of bites for which antivenins are available.

    a. _____

    b. _____

    c. _____

    d. _____

    e. _____

5. List four types of patients who should not be given human immune globulin intravenous products.

    a. _____

    b. _____

    c. _____

    d. _____

XIII. CLINICAL APPLICATION

1. Mrs. C has been exposed to the hepatitis B virus by her husband and has been given Nabi-HB. Explain to Mrs. C the most common adverse reactions of immune globulin therapy.

28 Antineoplastic Drugs

I. MATCHING

Match the term from Column A with the correct definition from Column B.

COLUMN A

_____ 1. alopecia

_____ 2. anemia

_____ 3. extravasation

_____ 4. leucopenia

_____ 5. stomatitis

_____ 6. thrombocytopenia

_____ 7. oral mucositis

_____ 8. vesicant

COLUMN B

A. Decrease in red blood cells.
B. Inflammation of the oral mucous membranes.
C. A decrease in the white blood cells or leukocytes.
D. Inflammation of the mouth.
E. An adverse drug reaction resulting in tissue necrosis.
F. Escape of fluid from a blood vessel into surrounding tissues.
G. The loss of hair.

II. MATCHING

Match the alkylating drug or antibiotic generic name in Column A with the correct trade name in Column B.

COLUMN A

_____ 1. epirubicin

_____ 2. cyclophosphamide

_____ 3. thiotepa

_____ 4. melphalan

_____ 5. iomustine

_____ 6. ifosfamide

_____ 7. chlorambucil

_____ 8. bleomycin sulfate

_____ 9. dactinomycin

_____ 10. idarubicin HCl

_____ 11. valrubicin

_____ 12. busulfan

COLUMN B

A. Thioplex
B. Idamycin
C. Cytoxan
D. Busulfex
E. Leukeran
F. Alkeran
G. Ifex
H. Ellence
I. Valstar
J. CeeNU
K. Cosmegen
L. Blenoxane

III. MATCHING

Match the generic antimetabolite or mitotic inhibitor in Column A with the correct trade name in Column B.

COLUMN A

_____ 1. paclitaxel

_____ 2. cladribine

_____ 3. cytarabine

_____ 4. vincristine sulfate

_____ 5. pentostatin

_____ 6. fludarabine

_____ 7. capecitabine

_____ 8. docetaxel

_____ 9. vinblastine sulfate

_____ 10. gemcitabine HCl

COLUMN B

A. Gemzar
B. Xeloda
C. Nipent
D. Cytosar-U
E. Oncovin
F. Fludara
G. Leustatin
H. Velban
I. Taxotere
J. Taxol

IV. MATCHING

Match the generic androgen, antiandrogen, progestin, estrogen, antiestrogen, or gonadotropin-releasing hormone analog in Column A to the correct trade name in Column B.

COLUMN A

_____ 1. toremifene citrate

_____ 2. nilutamide

_____ 3. goserelin acetate

_____ 4. diethylstilbestrol

_____ 5. tamoxifen citrate

_____ 6. leuprolide acetate

_____ 7. bicalutamide

_____ 8. triptorelin pamoate

_____ 9. estramustine

_____ 10. medroxyprogesterone

COLUMN B

A. Stilphostrol
B. Fareston
C. Zoladex
D. Casodex
E. Nolvadex
F. Emcyt
G. Lupron
H. Trelstar Depot
I. Depo-Provera
J. Nilandron

V. MATCHING

Match the generic aromatase inhibitor, epipodophyllotoxin, enzyme, platinum coordination complex, anthracenedione, or substituted urea in Column A with the correct trade name in Column B.

COLUMN A

_____ 1. teniposide (VM-26)

_____ 2. carboplatin

_____ 3. letrozole

_____ 4. etoposide

_____ 5. asparaginase

_____ 6. pegaspargase

_____ 7. hydroxyurea

_____ 8. cisplatin

_____ 9. mitoxantrone HCl

_____ 10. anastrazole

COLUMN B

A. Elspar
B. Femara
C. Platinol-AQ
D. Novantrone
E. Droxia
F. Paraplatin
G. Arimidex
H. Vumon
I. Toposar
J. Oncaspar

VI. MATCHING

Match the generic cytoprotective agent, DNA topoisomerase inhibitor, biological response modifier, retinoid, or rexinoid in Column A to the correct trade name in Column B.

COLUMN A

_____ 1. irinotecan HCl

_____ 2. bexarotene

_____ 3. dexrazoxane

_____ 4. topotecan HCl

_____ 5. aldesleukin

_____ 6. amifostine

_____ 7. tretinoin

_____ 8. levamisole

_____ 9. denileukin diftitox

_____ 10. BCG, intravesical

COLUMN B

A. Targretin
B. Proleukin
C. Hycamtin
D. Ontak
E. Zinecard
F. Ethyol
G. Vesanoid
H. Ergamisol
I. Pacis
J. Camptosar

VII. MATCHING

Match the generic monoclonal antibody or unclassified antineoplastic drug in Column A with the correct trade name in Column B.

COLUMN A

_____ 1. trastuzumab

_____ 2. alemtuzumab

_____ 3. imatinib mesylate

_____ 4. mitotane

_____ 5. gemtuzumab ozogamicin

_____ 6. ibritumomab tiuxetan

_____ 7. porfimer sodium

COLUMN B

A. Gleevec
B. Herceptin
C. Lysodren
D. Photofrin
E. Mylotarg
F. Zevalin
G. Campath

VIII. MATCHING

Match the trade name in Column A to the drug type in Column B. You may use an answer more than once.

COLUMN A

_____ 1. Taxol

_____ 2. Xeloda

_____ 3. Matulane

_____ 4. Teslac

_____ 5. Blenoxane

_____ 6. Lupron

_____ 7. Vumon

_____ 8. Leukeran

_____ 9. Ergamisol

_____ 10. Nolvadex

_____ 11. Targretin

_____ 12. Ifex

COLUMN B

A. Alkylating drug
B. Antibiotic
C. Antimetabolite
D. Mitotic inhibitor
E. Hormone
F. Miscellaneous anticancer drug

IX. MATCHING

Match the drug in Column A to the use in Column B.

COLUMN A

_____ 1. Matulane

_____ 2. Leustatin

_____ 3. Droxia

_____ 4. DaunoXome

_____ 5. Photofrin

_____ 6. Myleran

_____ 7. CeeNU

_____ 8. Lysodren

_____ 9. Cosmegen

COLUMN B

A. Chronic myelogenous leukemia
B. Hairy cell leukemia
C. Hodgkin's disease
D. Melanoma
E. Esophageal cancer
F. Adrenal cortical carcinoma
G. Brain tumors
H. Kaposi's sarcoma
I. Wilms' tumor

X. TRUE/FALSE

Indicate whether each statement is True (T) or False (F).

_____ 1. Antineoplastic drugs always lead to a complete cure of the malignancy.

_____ 2. Chemotherapy refers to the use of antineoplastic drug therapy.

_____ 3. Antineoplastic drugs affect only the rapidly dividing cancer cells.

_____ 4. Alkylating drugs bind with DNA, causing breaks and thus preventing DNA replication.

_____ 5. Antineoplastic antibiotics have the same anti-infective ability as anti-infective antibiotics.

_____ 6. Methotrexate and fluorouracil are examples of antimetabolites.

_____ 7. Gonadotropin-releasing hormone analogs act by stimulating the anterior pituitary secretion of gonadotropins.

_____ 8. Single antineoplastic drugs often produce a better result than combination drug therapy.

_____ 9. An antiemetic can be given before administering an antineoplastic drug to help prevent nausea and vomiting.

_____ 10. All patients respond the same to antineoplastic drugs.

_____ 11. Doxorubicin can cause severe hair loss.

_____ 12. A patient who is experiencing nausea and vomiting as an adverse reaction should avoid greasy or fatty foods as well as unpleasant sights, smells, and tastes.

_____ 13. Extravasation of antineoplastic drugs has little effect on surrounding soft tissue.

_____ 14. Patients who are unable to communicate the pain they feel with extravasation are at greater risk.

_____ 15. Live virus vaccines generally produce an enhanced antibody production response when administered with fluorouracil or certain antineoplastic antibiotics.

_____ 16. Food decreases the absorption of fluorouracil.

_____ 17. Vitamin preparations containing folic acid may decrease the effects of methotrexate.

_____ 18. Bicalutamide may decrease the effect of oral anticoagulants.

_____ 19. Goserelin is administered subcutaneously into the soft tissue of the abdomen in a pellet form.

_____ 20. Green tea contains polyphenols or flavonoids.

XI. MULTIPLE CHOICE

Circle the letter of the best answer.

1. In which of the following areas are cells rapidly dividing and therefore may be affected by antineoplastic drug therapy?
   a. mouth
   b. gastrointestinal tract
   c. gonads
   d. bone marrow
   e. all of the answers are correct

2. According to the cell kill theory _____ .
   a. the first course of chemotherapy should kill 50% of the cancer cells
   b. the first course of chemotherapy should kill 80% of the cancer cells
   c. the first course of chemotherapy should kill 90% of the cancer cells
   d. the first course of chemotherapy should kill 100% of the cancer cells
   e. only one mega dose of an antineoplastic drug is needed to kill most types of cancer cells

3. All of the following are examples of alkylating drugs except _____ .
   a. bleomycin sulfate
   b. busulfan
   c. chlorambucil
   d. melphalan
   e. thiotepa

4. Antineoplastic antibiotics _____ .
   a. overstimulate cell growth causing cell death
   b. delay or inhibit cell division
   c. change the metabolism of the cell
   d. interfere with DNA and RNA synthesis
   e. answers b and d are correct

5. Antimetabolites work by ____ .
   a. inactivating enzymes
   b. altering the structure of DNA
   c. changing the DNA's ability to replicate
   d. all of the answers are correct
   e. answers b and c are correct

6. Cisplatin is an example of a(n) ____ drug.
   a. alkylating
   b. miscellaneous antineoplastic
   c. antimetabolite
   d. antineoplastic antibiotic
   e. antimitotic

7. Adverse reactions to antineoplastic drugs are ____ .
   a. sometimes dose dependent
   b. caused by the effect the drug has on many cells of the body
   c. of a wide variety
   d. sometimes desirable
   e. all of the answers are correct

8. Hyperuricemia may occur with ____ .
   a. melphalan
   b. mercaptopurine
   c. plicamycin
   d. answers a and b are correct
   e. all of the answers are correct

9. All of the following drugs except one cause gradual hair loss. Identify the exception.
   a. vinblastine
   b. vincristine
   c. etoposide
   d. bleomycin
   e. methotrexate

10. Bone marrow suppression as an adverse reaction to antineoplastic drug therapy can cause ____ .
    a. anemia
    b. thrombocytopenia
    c. leucopenia
    d. leukocytosis
    e. all of the answers are correct

11. All of the following are signs of extravasation except ____ .
    a. swelling
    b. stinging, burning, or pain at the injection site
    c. easy bruising
    d. redness
    e. lack of blood return

12. When cisplatin is used concurrently with ____, there is an increased risk of ototoxicity.
    a. antigout drugs
    b. cyclophosphamide
    c. loop diuretics
    d. aminoglycosides
    e. answers c and d are correct

13. Which of the following antineoplastic antibiotics can cause an increased risk of bleeding when administered with aspirin, warfarin, heparin, or NSAIDs?
    a. plicamycin
    b. bleomycin
    c. mitomycin
    d. dactinomycin
    e. mitoxantrone

14. Patients taking oral antidiabetic drugs along with a miscellaneous antineoplastic drug may have an increased risk of ____ .
    a. hyperglycemia
    b. hypoglycemia
    c. drug antagonism
    d. additive antineoplastic effects
    e. answers a and b are correct

15. Which of the following miscellaneous antineoplastic drugs may alter the drug response of anticoagulants?
    a. asparaginase
    b. pegaspargase
    c. aldesleukin
    d. etoposide
    e. levamisole

XII. RECALL FACTS

Indicate which of the following statements are Facts with an F. If the statement is not a fact, leave the line blank.

About Anorexia as an Adverse Reaction

____ 1. Is a rare adverse reaction.

____ 2. Is common with antineoplastic drug therapy.

____ 3. Three large meals are better tolerated.

____ 4. Small, frequent meals are better tolerated.

____ 5. Breakfast is often the best tolerated meal.

____ 6. Lunch is often the best tolerated meal.

_____ 7. Nutritional supplements may be pre-scribed.

_____ 8. Patient's body weight is monitored weekly.

_____ 9. Patient's body weight is monitored monthly.

About Patients in Whom Antineoplastic Drugs Are Contraindicated

_____ 1. Leukopenia or thrombocytopenia

_____ 2. Polycythemia

_____ 3. Serious infections

_____ 4. Anemia

_____ 5. Serious renal disease

_____ 6. Obesity

_____ 7. Pregnancy

_____ 8. Those who work with children

About Pregnancy Category X Drugs

_____ 1. levamisole

_____ 2. goserelin

_____ 3. triptorelin

_____ 4. thioguanine

_____ 5. plicamycin

_____ 6. flutamide

_____ 7. bicalutamide

_____ 8. methotrexate

_____ 9. vinblastine

_____ 10. dactinomycin

_____ 11. diethylstilbestrol

XIII. FILL IN THE BLANK

Fill in the blanks using words from the list below.

intravenous   fluorouracil
earlier   antigout
less   tamoxifen
additive   stomatitis
temporary   antineoplastic
antimetabolites   mitotic inhibitor
treatment plan   alopecia
alkylating   dividing
gonadotropin-releasing
hormone analogs

1. _____ drugs can be used to cure, to control, or to provide palliative therapy of malignant tumors.

2. Chemotherapy is administered at the time the cell population is _____ to optimize cell death.

3. _____ drugs interfere with the process of cell division of both normal and malignant cells.

4. _____ disrupt normal cell functions by interfering with cellular metabolic functions.

5. _____ are used in the treatment of advanced prostatic carcinomas.

6. Vincristine is an example of a(n) _____ .

7. A(n) _____ for antineoplastic drug therapy can prevent, lessen, or treat most of the symptoms of a specific adverse reaction.

8. _____ may affect a patient's mental health.

9. Hair loss from antineoplastic drug therapy is _____ .

10. _____ or oral mucositis may occur 5–7 days after chemotherapy and continue up to 10 days after therapy.

11. The _____ extravasation is detected, the _____ likely soft-tissue damage will occur.

12. _____ is not compatible with diazepam, doxorubicin, or methotrexate.

13. Antimetabolite and alkylating agents may antagonize _____ drugs by increasing serum uric acid levels.

14. Estrogens decrease the effectiveness of

_____ .

15. _____ bone marrow depressive effects occur when a mitotic inhibitor drug is administered with another antineoplastic drug.

16. The most common and reliable route of drug delivery is the _____ route.

XIV. LIST

List the requested number of items.

1. List five antineoplastic antibiotics.

    a. _____

    b. _____

    c. _____

    d. _____

    e. _____

2. List six common adverse reactions of antineoplastic drugs.

    a. _____

    b. _____

    c. _____

    d. _____

    e. _____

    f. _____

3. List four symptoms that indicate thrombocytopenia.

    a. _____

    b. _____

    c. _____

    d. _____

4. List three examples of vesicant drugs.

    a. _____

    b. _____

    c. _____

5. List five things that a patient should be assessed for following the administration of an antineoplastic drug.

    a. _____

    b. _____

    c. _____

    d. _____

    e. _____

6. List three antineoplastic drugs that are administered orally.

    a. _____

    b. _____

    c. _____

7. List five beneficial effects of green tea.

    a. _____

    b. _____

    c. _____

    d. _____

    e. _____

XV. CLINICAL APPLICATIONS

1. Mr. Y was recently diagnosed with esophageal cancer. His healthcare provider has chosen porfimer sodium (Photofrin) as part of his antineoplastic drug therapy. What adverse reactions might Mr. Y experience while receiving this medication?

2. Explain to Miss P's family the six basic different types of drugs that may be used to treat her breast cancer and how each will help Miss P to get better.

29 Drugs That Affect the Musculoskeletal System

I. MATCHING

Match the term from Column A with the correct definition from Column B.

COLUMN A

_____ 1. chrysiasis

_____ 2. corticosteroids

_____ 3. gout

_____ 4. musculoskeletal

_____ 5. osteoarthritis

_____ 6. rheumatoid arthritis

COLUMN B

A. Grey to blue pigmentation of the skin that may occur from gold deposits in tissues.

B. A noninflammatory joint disease resulting in degeneration of the articular cartilage and changes in the synovial membrane.

C. The bone and muscular structure of the body.

D. A chronic disease characterized by inflammatory changes within the body's connective tissue.

E. A form of arthritis in which uric acid accumulates in increased amounts in the blood and often is deposited in the joints.

F. Hormones secreted from the adrenal cortex that contain potent anti-inflammatory action.

II. MATCHING

Match the generic drug name in Column A to the correct trade name in Column B.

COLUMN A

_____ 1. allopurinol

_____ 2. methocarbamol

_____ 3. cyclobenzaprine hydrochloride

_____ 4. leflunomide

_____ 5. gold sodium, thiomalate

_____ 6. probenecid

_____ 7. risedronate sodium

_____ 8. alendronate sodium

_____ 9. baclofen

_____ 10. penicillamine

_____ 11. chlorphenesin carbamate

_____ 12. prednisone

COLUMN B

A. Aurolate
B. Maolate
C. Flexeril
D. Deltasone
E. Robaxin
F. Fosamax
G. Arava
H. Zyloprim
I. Cuprimine
J. Benemid
K. Actonel
L. Lioresal

III. MATCHING

Match the generic or trade name in Column A to the type of drug in Column B. You may use an answer more than once.

COLUMN A

_____ 1. Enbrel

_____ 2. Didronel

_____ 3. Soma

_____ 4. Azulfidine

_____ 5. Solganal

_____ 6. Dantrium

_____ 7. Plaquenil sulfate

_____ 8. Synvisc

_____ 9. colchicines

_____ 10. sulfinpyrazone

_____ 11. Delta-Cortef

_____ 12. Banflex

COLUMN B

A. Drugs used to treat osteoporosis
B. Drugs used to treat gout
C. Skeletal muscle relaxants
D. Corticosteroids
E. Miscellaneous drugs

IV. MATCHING

Match the generic drug name in Column A with the correct use in Column B. You may use an answer more than once.

COLUMN A

_____ 1. probenecid

_____ 2. dantrolene sodium

_____ 3. etidronate

_____ 4. prednisone

_____ 5. aurothioglucose

_____ 6. auranofin

_____ 7. orphenadrine citrate

_____ 8. baclofen

_____ 9. etanercept

_____ 10. sulfasalazine

_____ 11. sulfinpyrazone

_____ 12. leflunomide

COLUMN B

A. Paget's disease
B. Rheumatoid arthritis
C. Gouty arthritis
D. Ankylosing spondylitis
E. Spasticity due to spinal cord injury
F. Discomfort due to musculoskeletal disorders

V. TRUE/FALSE

Indicate whether each statement is True (T) or False (F).

_____ 1. Gold compounds suppress or prevent arthritis and synovitis.

_____ 2. Gold compounds can reverse structural changes to the joints.

_____ 3. A metallic taste may occur before stomatitis becomes evident when gold compounds are used.

_____ 4. Thrombocytopenia can occur with gold compound therapy.

_____ 5. Zyloprim acts by dissolving urate crystals in the joints.

_____ 6. Drugs used to treat gout are used to manage acute attacks or to prevent acute attacks.

_____ 7. Benemid works by increasing the excretion of uric acid by the kidneys.

_____ 8. Patients being treated for gout should increase their fluid intake to approximately 3,000 mL/day.

_____ 9. Administration of allopurinol with aluminum salts may decrease the effectiveness of allopurinol.

_____ 10. Salicylates accelerate probenecid's uricosuric action.

_____ 11. There is a decreased incidence of skin rash when allopurinol and ampicillin are administered concurrently.

_____ 12. When a skeletal muscle relaxant is administered with alcohol, there is an increased CNS depressant effect.

_____ 13. Patients receiving hormone replacement therapy should not take bisphosphonates.

_____ 14. Alendronate bioavailability is increased when administered with ranitidine.

_____ 15. Absorption of bisphosphonates is increased when administered with calcium supplements or antacids.

_____ 16. Many adverse reactions are associated with high-dose and long-term corticosteroid therapy.

_____ 17. Any patient complaint related to penicillamine should be reported to the healthcare provider.

_____ 18. Any adverse reaction to hydroxychloroquine should immediately be reported to the healthcare provider.

_____ 19. Methotrexate is a Pregnancy Category X drug.

_____ 20. Patients who are allergic to penicillin can generally take penicillamine with no problems.

_____ 21. A total of 90–98% of the chondroitin molecules are absorbed.

_____ 22. Oral glucosamine theoretically provides a building block for regeneration of damaged cartilage.

_____ 23. No adverse reactions have been reported with glucosamine use.

_____ 24. Glucosamine and chondroitin are used to treat osteoarthritis.

_____ 25. Chondroitin molecules are large and therefore easily absorbed.

VI. MULTIPLE CHOICE

Circle the letter of the best answer.

1. Gold compound's _____ .
   a. effects occur slowly
   b. mechanism of action is unknown
   c. adverse reactions may occur many months after therapy has been discontinued
   d. answers a and c are correct
   e. all of the answers are correct

2. Chrysiasis _____ .
   a. is caused by gold deposits in tissues
   b. is a reaction that causes gold crystal to form in the joints
   c. is the result of too large of a dose of a gold compound
   d. only occurs with auranofin
   e. is a gold pigmentation of the sclera

3. Which of the following treatments for gout work by reducing the production of uric acid?
   a. colchicine
   b. allopurinol
   c. sulfinpyrazone
   d. probenecid
   e. aurothioglucose

4. Which of the drugs for gout are contraindicated in patients with peptic ulcer disease?
   a. gold compounds
   b. colchicines
   c. allopurinol
   d. sulfinpyrazone
   e. probenecid

5. _____ has an effect on muscle tone; therefore, it reduces muscle spasms.
   a. Soma
   b. Lioresal
   c. Flexeril
   d. Paraflex
   e. Valium

6. The most common adverse reaction of skeletal muscle relaxants is _____ .
   a. gastrointestinal distress
   b. drowsiness
   c. skin rash
   d. ototoxicity
   e. hepatitis

7. The skeletal muscle relaxant that is contraindicated in patients with a recent myocardial infarction is _____ .
   a. Baclofen
   b. Carisoprodol
   c. Cyclobenzaprine
   d. Dantrolene
   e. Meprobamate

8. Which bisphosphonate acts by inhibiting normal and abnormal bone resorption?
   a. alendronate
   b. etidronate
   c. risedronate
   d. answers b and c are correct
   e. all of the answers are correct

9. _____ is used for postoperative treatment after total hip replacement.
   a. Alendronate
   b. Etidronate
   c. Risedronate
   d. Answers b and c are correct
   e. All of the answers are correct

10. The mechanism of action of _____ is unknown in the treatment of rheumatoid arthritis.
    a. penicillamine
    b. methotrexate
    c. hydroxychloroquine
    d. answers a and c are correct
    e. all of the answers are correct

11. Which of the following drugs are used to treat rheumatoid arthritis in patients who have had an insufficient therapeutic response to other antirheumatic drugs?
    a. penicillamine
    b. methotrexate

c. hydroxychloroquine
d. answers a and c are correct
e. all of the answers are correct

12. _____ may have adverse effects on the eye as well as hematological effects.
   a. Penicillamine
   b. Methotrexate
   c. Hydroxychloroquine
   d. Allopurinol
   e. Baclofen

13. _____ may cause an increase in skin friability.
   a. Penicillamine
   b. Methotrexate
   c. Hydroxychloroquine
   d. Allopurinol
   e. Baclofen

14. _____ may cause abnormal hematology, liver function, or kidney function.
   a. Penicillamine
   b. Methotrexate
   c. Hydroxychloroquine
   d. Allopurinol
   e. Baclofen

15. Therapy with musculoskeletal drugs may _____ .
   a. keep the disorder under control
   b. improve the patient's daily living
   c. make the pain tolerable
   d. answers b and c are correct
   e. all of the answers are correct

16. Glucosamine _____ .
   a. is found in mucopolysaccharides, mucoproteins, and chitin
   b. is generally well tolerated
   c. is only used in combination with chondroitin
   d. answers a and b are correct
   e. all of the answers are correct

VII. FILL IN THE BLANK

Fill in the blanks using words from the list below.

decreases	skin rash
itching	unknown
bisphosphonates	hypocalcemia
90–98%	methotrexate
HylanG-F20	chondroitin
early	colchicine

1. The mechanism of action of gold compounds is _____ .

2. The greatest benefit of gold compounds appears to occur in patients in the _____ stages of disease.

3. _____ may occur before a skin reaction to gold compounds and should be reported immediately.

4. Tolerance for gold therapy _____ with advancing age.

5. _____ has no effect on uric acid metabolism.

6. Allopurinol has been associated with _____ as an adverse reaction.

7. _____ are used to treat Paget's disease.

8. Patients with _____ should not take alendronate or risedronate.

9. _____ is used to treat osteoarthritis knee pain and is administered directly into the knee.

10. _____ is used to treat severe disabling rheumatoid disease that is not responsive to other treatments.

11. _____ acts as the flexible connecting matrix between the protein filaments in cartilage.

12. Absorption of oral glucosamine is _____ .

VIII. CLINICAL APPLICATION

1. Mrs. L has been prescribed a bisphosphonate for her postmenopausal osteoporosis. The healthcare provider has asked you to tell her how best to take this type of drug. Give Mrs. L some advice about taking this medication.

30 Topical Drugs Used in the Treatment of Skin Disorders

I. MATCHING

Match the term from Column A with the correct definition from Column B.

COLUMN A

_____ 1. antipsoriatics

_____ 2. antiseptic

_____ 3. bactericidal

_____ 4. bacteriostatic

_____ 5. germicide

_____ 6. keratolytic

_____ 7. necrotic

_____ 8. proteolysis

_____ 9. purulent exudates

_____ 10. superinfection

COLUMN B

A. A drug that stops, slows, or prevents the growth of microorganisms.
B. A substance that destroys bacteria.
C. A drug that removes excess growth of the epidermis in disorders such as warts.
D. Drugs used to treat psoriasis.
E. Dead, as in dead tissue.
F. The slowing or retarding of the multiplication of bacteria.
G. An overgrowth of bacterial or fungal microorganisms not affected by the antibiotic being administered.
H. The process of hastening the reduction of proteins into simpler substances.
I. A drug that kills bacteria.
J. Pus-containing fluid.

II. MATCHING

Match the generic antibiotic or antipsoriatic drug name in Column A with the correct trade name in Column B.

COLUMN A

_____ 1. erythromycin

_____ 2. selenium sulfide

_____ 3. azelaic acid

_____ 4. benzoyl peroxide

_____ 5. gentamicin

_____ 6. metronidazole

_____ 7. sulfacetamide sodium

_____ 8. bacitracin

_____ 9. ammoniated mercury

_____ 10. anthralin

_____ 11. calcipotriene

_____ 12. mupirocin

COLUMN B

A. Emersal
B. Benzac
C. Sebizon
D. Miconal
E. Emgel
F. G-myticin
G. Bactroban
H. Baciguent
I. Dovonex
J. Metro-Gel
K. Azelex
L. Selsun Blue

III. MATCHING

Match the generic antifungal or antiviral drug in Column A with the trade name in Column B.

COLUMN A

_____ 1. haloprogin

_____ 2. penciclovir

_____ 3. oxiconazole

_____ 4. butenafine HCl

_____ 5. acyclovir

_____ 6. terbinafine HCl

_____ 7. sulconazole nitrate

_____ 8. ketoconazole

_____ 9. econazole nitrate

_____ 10. ciclopirox

_____ 11. amphotericin B

_____ 12. tolnaftate

COLUMN B

A. Zovirax
B. Mentax
C. Oxistat
D. Denavir
E. Spectazole
F. Loprox
G. Nizoral
H. Lamisil
I. Exelderm
J. Halotex
K. Tinactin
L. Fungizone

IV. MATCHING

Match the generic antiseptic/germicide, enzyme preparation, keratolytic, or local anesthetic drug in Column A to the correct trade name in Column B.

COLUMN A

_____ 1. triclosan

_____ 2. benzocaine

_____ 3. salicylic acid

_____ 4. povidone-iodine

_____ 5. lidocaine

_____ 6. chlorhexidine gluconate

_____ 7. masoprocol

_____ 8. collagenase

_____ 9. dibucaine

_____ 10. lidocaine HCl

_____ 11. benzalkonium chloride

_____ 12. diclofenac sodium

COLUMN B

A. Betadine
B. Santyl
C. Actinex
D. Betasept/Hibiclens
E. Xylocaine
F. Lanacane
G. Solaraze
H. Nupercainal
I. Benza
J. Duofilm
K. DentiPatch
L. Clearasil Daily Face Wash

V. MATCHING

Match the generic topical corticosteroid in Column A with the correct trade name in Column B.

COLUMN A

_____ 1. augmented betamethasone dipropionate

_____ 2. desoximetasone

_____ 3. triamcinolone acetonide

_____ 4. fluocinolone acetonide

_____ 5. amcinonide

_____ 6. hydrocortisone butyrate

_____ 7. alclometasone dipropionate

_____ 8. dexamethasone sodium phosphate

_____ 9. hydrocortisone buteprate

_____ 10. flurandrenolide

COLUMN B

A. Diprolene
B. Decadron Phosphate
C. Locoid
D. Fluonid
E. Kenalog
F. Pandel
G. Cordran
H. Aclovate
I. Cyclocort
J. Topicort

VI. MATCHING

Match the drug in Column A with the correct use in Column B.

COLUMN A

_____ 1. Denavir

_____ 2. Accuzyme

_____ 3. Metro-Gel

_____ 4. Xylocaine

_____ 5. Azelex

_____ 6. Halotex

_____ 7. Miconal

_____ 8. Solaraze

_____ 9. Bactroban

_____ 10. Betasept

COLUMN B

A. Acne vulgaris
B. Rosacea
C. Impetigo
D. Tinea pedis, tinea cruris
E. Herpes labialis
F. Surgical scrub
G. Psoriasis
H. Actinic keratoses
 I. Topical anesthesia
 J. Debridement of necrotic tissue

VII. TRUE/FALSE

Indicate whether each statement is True (T) or False (F).

_____ 1. Topical anti-infectives include antibiotics, antifungals, and antiviral drugs.

_____ 2. Topical antibiotics are only bacteriostatic.

_____ 3. Antifungal drugs work by inhibiting the growth of fungi.

_____ 4. Acyclovir is used as part of the initial treatment of genital warts.

_____ 5. There are no significant interactions with the topical anti-infectives.

_____ 6. An antiseptic works the same as a germicide.

_____ 7. Except for econazole nitrate and ciclopirox, the pregnancy categories of the antifungals are unknown.

_____ 8. Topical corticosteroids reduce itching, redness, and swelling when applied to inflamed skin.

_____ 9. Topical anti-psoriatics help remove the plaques associated with psoriasis.

_____ 10. Numbness and dermatitis may occur as adverse reactions of topical enzymes.

_____ 11. It is common practice to use topical enzymes to treat wounds in which nerves are exposed.

_____ 12. Keratolytics are used to remove warts, calluses, corns, and seborrheic keratoses.

_____ 13. Patients with diabetes or impaired circulation should not use keratolytics.

_____ 14. Topical anesthetics may be applied to the skin or mucous membranes.

_____ 15. Patients receiving Class I antiarrhythmic drugs should use tocainide cautiously.

_____ 16. Adults older than 65 years generally have fewer skin-related adverse reactions to calcipotriene than younger adults.

_____ 17. Aloe is used to prevent infection and promote healing of minor burns.

VIII. MULTIPLE CHOICE

Circle the letter of the best answer.

1. _____ is used to treat eczema.
   a. Fungizone
   b. Clioquinol
   c. Penciclovir
   d. Erythromycin
   e. Denavir

2. Which of the following is an example of a topical antibiotic?
   a. Micatin
   b. Zephiran
   c. Hibiclens
   d. Bacitracin
   e. Zovirax

3. The only topical antiviral drugs currently available besides Zovirax is _____ .
   a. penciclovir
   b. acyclovir
   c. ciclopirox
   d. amphotericin B
   e. chlorhexidine gluconate

4. Prolonged use of topical antibiotic preparations may result in a superficial _____ .
   a. hypersensitivity reaction
   b. rash
   c. superinfection
   d. viral infection
   e. none of the answers are correct

5. _____ toxicity can cause ototoxicity and nephrotoxicity.
   a. Acyclovir
   b. Econazole nitrate

c. Penciclovir
d. Ciclopirox
e. Neomycin

6. Topical corticosteroids vary in potency because
   of the _____ .
   a. concentration of the drug
   b. suspension vehicle
   c. area where the drug is applied
   d. answers a and c are correct
   e. all of the answers are correct

7. Which of the following is not a topical corticosteroid?
   a. Cyclocort
   b. Antra-Derm
   c. Diprosone
   d. Flurosyn
   e. Cort-Dome

8. Topical corticosteroids are contraindicated in
   which of the following situations?
   a. known hypersensitivity
   b. as monotherapy for bacterial skin infections
   c. for use on the face, groin, or axilla
   d. for ophthalmic use
   e. all of the answers are correct

9. Topical anesthetics _____ .
   a. may be applied to mucous membranes
   b. may be used to relieve itching and pain
      caused by skin conditions
   c. are commonly used for ophthalmic pur-
      poses
   d. answers a and b are correct
   e. all of the answers are correct

10. A patient who is using lidocaine viscous
    should not eat food for 1 hour after use be-
    cause _____ .
    a. they may have impaired swallowing abili-
       ties and may aspirate
    b. the food will decrease the activity of the an-
       esthetic
    c. the food will increase the absorption of the
       drug
    d. they will not be able to taste the food
    e. they may forget to chew

IX. RECALL FACTS

*Indicate which of the following statements are Facts
with an F. If the statement is not a fact, leave the
line blank.*

About Topical Antiseptics and Germicides

_____ 1. Chlorhexidine gluconate affects a wide
          range of microorganisms.

_____ 2. Hibiclens can affect Gram-negative and
          Gram-positive bacteria.

_____ 3. Benzalkonium solutions are bacterio-
          static.

_____ 4. Zephiran is active against bacteria, some
          viruses, fungi, and protozoa.

_____ 5. Povidone-iodine is less preferred than io-
          dine solution.

_____ 6. Povidone-iodine–treated areas may be
          bandaged.

_____ 7. Iodine is effective against many bacteria,
          fungi, viruses, yeasts, and protozoa.

_____ 8. Topical antiseptics and germicides are
          only used on skin surfaces.

_____ 9. Topical antiseptics and germicides have
          few adverse reactions.

_____ 10. Topical antiseptics and germicides have
          no significant precautions or interac-
          tions when used as directed.

X. FILL IN THE BLANK

Fill in the blanks using words from the list below.

hexachlorophene	synergistic
anthralin	C
aloe	keratolytics
topical enzymes	anti-inflammatory
bacteriostatic	discontinuing

1. _____ drugs work by slowing
   or retarding the multiplication of bacteria.

2. Topical antibiotics are Pregnancy Category
   _____ .

3. Topical corticosteroids exert localized
   _____ activity.

4. _____ may cause a temporary discoloration of the hair and fingernails.

5. _____ aid in the removal of dead soft tissue by hastening the reduction of proteins into smaller substances.

6. _____ may inhibit the activity of topical enzymes.

7. _____ are contraindicated for use on warts on mucous membranes.

8. Mexiletine and Class I antiarrhythmics have toxic effects which are potentially

_____ .

9. Adverse reactions caused by topical drugs can generally be relieved by _____ the drug.

10. _____ is an herb that helps repair skin tissue and reduce inflammation.

XI. LIST

List the requested number of items.

1. List three topical antifungal drugs used to treat tinea pedis, tinea cruris, tinea corporis, and superficial candidiasis.

   a. _____

   b. _____

   c. _____

2. List five adverse reactions to topical anti-infectives.

   a. _____

   b. _____

   c. _____

   d. _____

   e. _____

3. List five uses of topical corticosteroids.

   a. _____

   b. _____

   c. _____

   d. _____

   e. _____

4. List three conditions that may be treated with a topical enzyme.

   a. _____

   b. _____

   c. _____

5. List five uses of aloe.

   a. _____

   b. _____

   c. _____

   d. _____

   e. _____

XII. CLINICAL APPLICATION

1. Ms. G has been using a topical corticosteroid to help manage a skin condition. She has noted that the area seems to be dry and is itching more. What might Ms. G do to help relieve this adverse reaction to the medication?

31 Otic and Ophthalmic Preparations

I. MATCHING

Match the term from Column A with the correct definition from Column B.

COLUMN A

_____ 1. cycloplegia

_____ 2. miosis

_____ 3. miotic

_____ 4. mydriasis

_____ 5. mydriatics

_____ 6. otic

COLUMN B

A. Drugs that dilate the pupil, constrict superficial blood vessels of the sclera, and decrease the formation of aqueous humor.
B. Dilation of the pupil.
C. Paralysis of the ciliary muscle, resulting in an inability to focus the eye.
D. Ear.
E. Drugs used to help contract the pupil of the eye.
F. The contraction of the pupil of the eye.

II. MATCHING

Match the trade name of the otic preparation in Column A with the type of preparation in Column B. You may use an answer more than once.

COLUMN A

_____ 1. Ear-Eze

_____ 2. Chloromycetin Otic

_____ 3. Cortic

_____ 4. Otocort

_____ 5. Otomar-HC

_____ 6. Cipro HC Otic

_____ 7. Coly-Mycin S Otic

_____ 8. Otobiotic Otic

_____ 9. Cerumenex Drops

_____ 10. Auralgan Otic

COLUMN B

A. Steroid and antibiotic combination solutions
B. Steroid and antibiotic combinations, suspensions
C. Otic antibiotics
D. Select miscellaneous preparations

III. MATCHING

Match the generic ophthalmic drug name in Column A with the correct trade name in Column B.

COLUMN A

_____ 1. levobetaxolol HCl

_____ 2. carbachol

_____ 3. unoprostone isopropyl

_____ 4. ketorolac tromethamine

_____ 5. epinephrine

_____ 6. brinzolamide

_____ 7. pilocarpine nitrate

_____ 8. apraclonidine HCl

_____ 9. loteprednol etabonate

_____ 10. pemirolast potassium

_____ 11. carteolol HCl

_____ 12. idoxuridine

COLUMN B

A. Carboptic
B. Azopt
C. Epifrin
D. Alamast
E. Iopidine
F. Herplex
G. Ocupress
H. Betaxon
I. Pilagan
J. Rescula
K. Alrex
L. Acular

IV. MATCHING

Match the generic ophthalmic drug name in Column A with the correct trade name in Column B.

COLUMN A

_____ 1. dapiprazole HCl

_____ 2. glycerin, sodium chloride

_____ 3. natamycin

_____ 4. sodium sulfacetamide

_____ 5. atropine sulfate

_____ 6. prednisolone

_____ 7. brimonidine tartrate

_____ 8. fluorometholone

_____ 9. oxymetazoline hydrochloride

_____ 10. erythromycin

COLUMN B

A. Natacyn
B. Eye-Lube-A
C. AK-Sulf
D. Flarex
E. Isopto-Atropine
F. Ilotycin
G. Visine L.R.
H. AK-Pred
I. Alphagan
J. Rev-Eyes

V. MATCHING

Match the ophthalmic preparation trade name in Column A with the type of preparation in Column B.

COLUMN A

_____ 1. Pilagan

_____ 2. Tobrex

_____ 3. Isopto Homatropine

_____ 4. Maxidex

_____ 5. Ocupress

_____ 6. Rev-Eyes

_____ 7. Voltaren

_____ 8. Humorsol

_____ 9. Visine

_____ 10. Propine

_____ 11. AK-Sulf

_____ 12. Alocril

_____ 13. Alphagan

_____ 14. Lumigan

_____ 15. Vira-A

_____ 16. Trusopt

_____ 17. Natacyn

COLUMN B

A. Alpha$_2$-adrenergic agonist
B. Sympathomimetics
C. Alpha-adrenergic blocking drugs
D. Beta-adrenergic blocking drugs
E. Miotics, direct acting
F. Miotics, cholinesterase inhibitors
G. Carbonic anhydrase inhibitors
H. Prostaglandin agonist
I. Mast cell stabilizer
J. NSAID
K. Corticosteroids
L. Antibiotics
M. Sulfonamides
N. Antiviral drugs
O. Antifungal drugs
P. Vasoconstrictors/mydriatics
Q. Cycloplegic/mydriatics

VI. MATCHING

Match the ophthalmic preparation in Column A with the correct use in Column B.

COLUMN A

_____ 1. Humorsol

_____ 2. silver nitrate

_____ 3. Alrex

_____ 4. Betoptic

_____ 5. Ocufen

_____ 6. Natacyn

_____ 7. echothiophate iodide

_____ 8. E-Pilo-1

_____ 9. Vira-A

_____ 10. Garamycin

COLUMN B

A. Treatment of fungal eye infections
B. Prevention of ophthalmia neonatorum
C. Treatment of eye infections
D. Allergic conjunctivitis
E. Glaucoma
F. Treatment of herpes simplex keratitis
G. Chronic open-angle glaucoma
H. Elevated IOP
I. Glaucoma and strabismus
J. Inhibition of intraoperative miosis

VII. TRUE/FALSE

Indicate whether each statement is True (T) or False (F).

_____ 1. Miscellaneous preparations for the treatment of otic conditions may contain antipyrine.

_____ 2. Otic preparations are used to treat inner ear infections.

_____ 3. It is safe to use drugs to remove cerumen at any time.

_____ 4. No significant drug interactions have been reported with the use of otic preparations.

_____ 5. The incidence of adverse reactions associated with ophthalmic drugs is usually small.

_____ 6. Brimonidine tartrate is used to treat open-angle glaucoma or ocular hypertension.

_____ 7. Sympathomimetic drugs lower intraocular pressure by increasing the outflow of aqueous humor in the eye.

_____ 8. Systemic reactions never occur with sympathomimetic drugs used to treat ocular conditions.

_____ 9. When beta-adrenergic drugs for ophthalmic purposes are administered with oral beta blockers there may be an increased or additive effect of the drugs.

_____ 10. Cholinesterase inhibitors cause an increased resistance to aqueous flow.

_____ 11. Systemic toxicity (i.e., nausea, vomiting, diarrhea) occurs more often with cholinesterase inhibitors than with miotics.

_____ 12. Carbonic anhydrase inhibitors are used in the treatment of elevated intraocular pressure seen in open-angle glaucoma.

_____ 13. Carbonic anhydrase inhibitors are contraindicated during pregnancy and lactation.

_____ 14. Prostaglandin agonists are contraindicated during pregnancy.

_____ 15. Mast cell stabilizers work by stimulating the release of anti-inflammatory mediators.

_____ 16. Ketorolac is a nonsteroidal anti-inflammatory drug used for the relief of itching of eyes caused by seasonal allergies.

_____ 17. A patient who has had a superficial corneal foreign body should not be given a corticosteroidal ophthalmic preparation.

_____ 18. Antiviral drugs interfere with viral metabolism processes.

_____ 19. Antifungal drugs can act against yeast.

_____ 20. Systemic adverse reactions of ophthalmic vasoconstrictors and mydriatics can include headaches, tachycardia, and stroke.

_____ 21. Cycloplegic mydriatics cause paralysis of the ciliary muscle.

_____ 22. Cycloplegic mydriatics have had no significant drug interactions reported when the drugs are given topically.

_____ 23. Bilberry is given as an antioxidant.

VIII. MULTIPLE CHOICE

Circle the letter of the best answer.

1. Carbamide peroxide found in miscellaneous otic preparations is used to _____ .
   a. provide antifungal action
   b. provide analgesia
   c. prevent inflammation
   d. help remove ear wax
   e. produce local anesthesia

2. Ophthalmic preparations may be used for _____ .
   a. lowering intraocular pressure
   b. bacterial or viral infections
   c. inflammatory conditions
   d. symptoms of allergy related to the eye
   e. all of the answers are correct

3. _____ is an alpha$_2$-adrenergic receptor agonist.
   a. Apraclonidine
   b. Brimonidine tartrate
   c. Epinephrine
   d. Dipivefrin
   e. Dapiprazole

4. Patients taking _____ should not use brimonidine tartrate.

    a. oral contraceptives
    b. estrogen replacement therapy
    c. monoamine oxidase inhibitors
    d. antibiotics
    e. oral anticoagulants

5. _____ is used to control or prevent postoperative elevations in intraocular pressure.

    a. Apraclonidine
    b. Brimonidine tartrate
    c. Dapiprazole
    d. Dorzolamide
    e. Ketorolac

6. Epinephrine should not be used while wearing soft contact lenses because _____ .

    a. it changes the shape of the lens
    b. it causes clouding of the lens
    c. it results in an inflammatory reaction
    d. discoloration of the lenses may occur
    e. it prevents gas exchange

7. Dapiprazole is used to _____ .

    a. reverse diagnostic mydriasis
    b. block the beta-adrenergic receptors causing dilation of the iris
    c. inhibit narrow-angle glaucoma
    d. reduce the production of tears
    e. none of the answers are correct

8. In which of the following conditions are beta-adrenergic blocking drugs contraindicated?

    a. acute iritis
    b. pregnancy
    c. sinus bradycardia
    d. conjunctivitis
    e. ptosis

9. Cholinesterase inhibitors are used to treat _____ .

    a. open-angle glaucoma
    b. closed-angle glaucoma
    c. iritis
    d. conjunctivitis
    e. retinal detachment

10. Iris cysts may form in patients taking cholinesterase inhibitors but will usually shrink _____ .

    a. after discontinuation of the drug
    b. after a reduction in frequency of instillation
    c. after a reduction in strength of the drops
    d. all of the answers are correct
    e. none of the answers are correct; iris cysts are permanent

11. Prostaglandin agonists are used _____ .

    a. to lower intraocular pressure
    b. to raise intraocular pressure
    c. to increase the flow of aqueous humor out of the eye
    d. answers a and b are correct
    e. answers a and c are correct

12. Mast cell stabilizers are used for _____ .

    a. blurred vision correction
    b. the prevention of eye itching caused by allergic conjunctivitis
    c. lowering intraocular pressure
    d. treatment of macular degeneration
    e. treatment of night blindness

13. In which patient is the use of a mast cell stabilizer contraindicated?

    a. A patient who wears colored contact lenses.
    b. A patient with open-angle glaucoma.
    c. A patient with a hypersensitivity to the medication.
    d. Answers a and c are correct
    e. All of the answers are correct

14. Which nonsteroidal anti-inflammatory drug might be chosen to prevent miosis during eye surgery?

    a. diclofenac
    b. ketorolac
    c. nedocromil
    d. flurbiprofen
    e. pemirolast

15. Nonsteroidal anti-inflammatory drugs used for ophthalmic purposes have as their most common adverse reaction _____ .

    a. transient burning and stinging
    b. discoloration of contact lenses
    c. increased intraocular pressures
    d. iritis
    e. dry eyes

16. Which of the following are potential adverse reactions of corticosteroid use?

    a. elevated intraocular pressure
    b. loss of visual acuity
    c. cataract formation
    d. delayed wound healing
    e. all of the answers are correct

17. Vasoconstrictors and mydriatics can act to _____ .

    a. dilate the pupil
    b. constrict superficial blood vessels of the sclera

c. decrease the formation of aqueous humor
d. answers a and b are correct
e. all of the answers are correct

18. A patient needing to have his or her pupils dilated for examination of the eye may be given a _____ .
  a. vasoconstrictor
  b. nonsteroidal anti-inflammatory drug
  c. corticosteroid
  d. mydriatic
  e. miotic

19. Vasoconstrictors and mydriatics would be contraindicated in a patient with _____ .
  a. sulfite sensitivity
  b. iritis
  c. narrow-angle glaucoma
  d. answers a and c are correct
  e. answers a and b are correct

20. Cycloplegic mydriatics are used _____ .
  a. to treat inflammatory conditions of the iris
  b. to treat inflammatory conditions of the uveal tract
  c. for examination of the eye
  d. none of the answers are correct
  e. all of the answers are correct

21. Inactive ingredients in artificial tears may include which of the following?
  a. preservatives
  b. antioxidants
  c. drugs that slow drainage
  d. answers a and c are correct
  e. all of the answers are correct

22. Bilberry _____ .
  a. promotes cone bleaching in the retina
  b. allows red blood cells to shrink
  c. increases the production of enzymes in the eye
  d. keeps hands and feet capillaries from dilating
  e. none of the answers are correct

IX. RECALL FACTS

Indicate which of the following statements are Facts with an F. If the statement is not a fact, leave the line blank.

About Antibiotics, Sulfonamides, and Silver

_____ 1. Antibiotics have antibacterial activity.

_____ 2. Sulfonamides are effective only against Gram-positive microorganisms.

_____ 3. Silver possesses antibacterial activity against both Gram-positive and Gram-negative microorganisms.

_____ 4. Antibiotics are used to treat corneal ulcers.

_____ 5. Sulfonamides are used in the treatment of conjunctivitis.

_____ 6. Silver nitrate can be used to prevent gonorrheal ophthalmia neonatorum.

_____ 7. Tetracycline and erythromycin can be used to treat gonorrheal ophthalmia neonatorum.

_____ 8. Patients with epithelial herpes simplex are commonly treated with sulfonamide ophthalmics.

About Patient Management Issues with Ophthalmic Preparations

_____ 1. Ophthalmic ointments are applied to the eyelids or dropped into the lower conjunctival sac.

_____ 2. Ophthalmic solutions are applied under the eyelid.

_____ 3. When applying two eye drop prescriptions at the same time, wait at least 5 minutes before instilling the second drug.

_____ 4. Ophthalmic drugs may produce blurred vision.

_____ 5. Any liquid medication can be applied to the eye.

_____ 6. Sympathomimetic ophthalmic drugs can cause systemic effects in patients.

_____ 7. Visual impairment caused by ophthalmic drugs never lasts more than 30 minutes.

_____ 8. Ophthalmic drug containers can be warmed in the hands before instilling the drug.

X. FILL IN THE BLANK

Fill in the blanks using words from the list below.

miotics	adrenochrome
impaired	respiratory tract
prostaglandin	natamycin
mydriatics	artificial tear
systemically	nedocromil
pemirolast	diclofenac
corticosteroids	superinfection
reducing	dipivefrin

1. Prolonged use of otic preparations containing an antibiotic may result in a(n)

   _____ .

2. Patients using otic preparations should be told that hearing in the treated ear may be

   _____ while the solution remains in the ear canal.

3. Brimonidine tartrate works by

   _____ aqueous humor production.

4. Prolonged use of sympathomimetic drugs for treatment of ocular disorders may result in

   _____ deposits in the cornea and conjunctiva.

5. _____ appears to be better tolerated and has fewer adverse reactions than other sympathomimetic drugs used to lower intraocular pressure.

6. _____ contract the pupil of the eye.

7. Persons working with insecticides containing carbamate or organophosphate are at risk for systemic effects of cholinesterase inhibitors because of absorption through the

   _____ or the skin.

8. Most carbonic anhydrase inhibitors are administered _____ .

9. Mast cell stabilizers currently used for ophthalmic use are _____ and

   _____ .

10. _____ can be used to treat postoperative inflammation after eye surgery.

11. Nonsteroidal anti-inflammatory drugs work by inhibiting _____ synthesis.

12. Prolonged use of _____ may result in elevated intraocular pressure and nerve damage.

13. _____ is the only ophthalmic antifungal drug in use.

14. Exaggerated adrenergic effects may occur when _____ are administered with MAOIs.

15. _____ solutions lubricate the eyes and can be used to treat dry eyes.

XI. LIST

List the requested number of items.

1. List the five ingredients and percentages found in Acetasol HC.
   a. _____
   b. _____
   c. _____
   d. _____
   e. _____

2. List the three categories of otic preparations.
   a. _____
   b. _____
   c. _____

3. List four uses of otic preparations.
   a. _____
   b. _____
   c. _____
   d. _____

4. List four conditions in which drugs to remove cerumen should not be used.
   a. _____
   b. _____

c. _____

d. _____

5. List five transient local reactions to sympatho-mimetic drugs.

a. _____

b. _____

c. _____

d. _____

e. _____

6. List five adverse reactions of dapiprazole.

a. _____

b. _____

c. _____

d. _____

e. _____

7. List five conditions in which miotics are used with caution.

a. _____

b. _____

c. _____

d. _____

e. _____

8. List five ophthalmic uses of corticosteroids.

a. _____

b. _____

c. _____

d. _____

e. _____

9. List three uses of antiviral drugs in ophthalmic disorders.

a. _____

b. _____

c. _____

10. List five systemic adverse reactions of cycloplegic mydriatics.

a. _____

b. _____

c. _____

d. _____

e. _____

11. List four other names for bilberry.

a. _____

b. _____

c. _____

d. _____

XII. CLINICAL APPLICATION

1. Mrs. P, age 76, has been to see her healthcare provider to be treated for pain and irritation in her external auditory canal. After determining that there is no infection at the site, her healthcare provider decides to prescribe medication to help ease her discomfort. Using the Summary Drug Table of Otic Preparations, choose a medication that will be effective and easy for her to instill by herself.

2. Mr. H, age 82, has been diagnosed with glaucoma. He is also currently taking a beta blocker for cardiac problems. Given his medical history, which of the sympathomimetic ophthalmic preparations would be the best choice for his glaucoma treatment regimen?

32 Fluids and Electrolytes

I. MATCHING

Match the term from Column A with the correct definition from Column B.

COLUMN A

_____ 1. electrolyte

_____ 2. extravasation

_____ 3. half-normal saline

_____ 4. hypocalcemia

_____ 5. hypokalemia

_____ 6. hyponatremia

_____ 7. normal saline

_____ 8. protein substrates

COLUMN B

A. An electrically charged particle that is essential for normal cell function and is involved in various metabolic activities.
B. Low blood calcium.
C. Solution containing 0.45% NaCl.
D. Solution containing 0.9% NaCl.
E. Escape of fluid from a vessel into surrounding tissues.
F. Amino acid preparations that act to promote the production of proteins and are essential to life.
G. Low blood sodium.
H. Low blood potassium.

II. MATCHING

Match the generic electrolyte name in Column A with the correct trade name in Column B.

COLUMN A

_____ 1. calcium citrate

_____ 2. magnesium

_____ 3. potassium replacements

_____ 4. calcium lactate oral electrolyte mixture

_____ 5. calcium carbonate

_____ 6. calcium acetate

COLUMN B

A. Pedialyte
B. Effer K
C. PhosLo
D. Almora
E. Tums EX
F. Citracal

III. MATCHING

Match the electrolyte imbalance in Column A with the signs and symptoms in Column B.

COLUMN A

_____ 1. hypocalcemia

_____ 2. hypercalcemia

_____ 3. hypomagnesemia

_____ 4. hypermagnesemia

_____ 5. hypokalemia

_____ 6. hyperkalemia

_____ 7. hyponatremia

_____ 8. hypernatremia

COLUMN B

A. Anorexia, nausea, vomiting, ECG changes
B. Leg and foot cramps, hypertension, tachycardia
C. Lethargy, drowsiness, impaired respiration
D. Fever, hot-dry skin, dry, sticky mucous membranes
E. Hyperactive reflexes, muscle twitching, muscle cramps, tetany
F. Cold, clammy skin, decreased skin turgor, apprehension
G. Irritability, anxiety, listlessness, mental confusion
H. Anorexia, nausea, bone tenderness, polyuria, polydipsia, cardiac arrest

IV. MATCHING

Match the information in Column A with the correct electrolyte in Column B. You may use and answer more than once.

COLUMN A

_____ 1. used in the treatment of metabolic acidosis

_____ 2. is important in the transmission of nerve impulses

_____ 3. used for blood clotting and bone and teeth building

_____ 4. contraction of smooth, cardiac, and skeletal muscles

_____ 5. used as a gastric and urinary alkalinizer

_____ 6. may decrease the absorption of ketoconazole

_____ 7. used in the treatment of hypocalcemia

_____ 8. used to treat hypokalemia

_____ 9. maintenance of normal heart action

_____ 10. used in half-normal and normal saline

_____ 11. can cause local tissue necrosis if extravasation occurs

_____ 12. is contraindicated in patients with hypercalcemia, with ventricular fibrillation, or who are taking digitalis

COLUMN B

A. Bicarbonate
B. Calcium
C. Magnesium
D. Potassium
E. Sodium

V. TRUE/FALSE

Indicate whether each statement is True (T) or False (F).

_____ 1. No interactions have been reported in the use of blood plasma.

_____ 2. Plasma protein fractions are administered intramuscularly.

_____ 3. A blood type and cross-match are not needed when plasma protein fractions are given.

_____ 4. Protein substrates have no known adverse reactions.

_____ 5. Energy substrates include dextrose solutions and fat emulsions.

_____ 6. No more than 60% of a patient's total caloric intake should come from fat emulsion.

_____ 7. Fat emulsions are used in patients requiring parenteral nutrition for extended periods.

_____ 8. Plasma expanders can be used as a substitute for whole blood or plasma in the treatment of shock.

_____ 9. Fat solution infusion patients should be carefully observed during the first 30 minutes of infusion for signs of a reaction.

_____ 10. Frequent serum electrolyte levels should be used to monitor electrolyte therapy.

_____ 11. Peripheral total parenteral nutrition is used in patients who are severely hypercatabolic.

_____ 12. Hyperglycemia is the most common metabolic complication of total parenteral nutrition.

VI. MULTIPLE CHOICE

Circle the letter of the best answer.

1. Human plasma is used to _____ .
   a. replace red blood cell volume
   b. increase blood volume
   c. replace plasma proteins
   d. restore electrolyte balance
   e. protect against transfusion reactions

2. Serum albumin _____ .
   a. is obtained from donated whole blood
   b. is a protein found in plasma
   c. can be artificially produced
   d. answers a and b are correct
   e. answers b and c are correct

3. Plasma protein fractions are used to treat _____ .
   a. hypervolemic shock
   b. hypovolemic shock
   c. hypoproteinemia
   d. answers a and c are correct
   e. answers b and c are correct

4. Protein substrates _____ .

   a. are amino acid preparations that act to promote the production of proteins
   b. are commonly given to treat kidney failure
   c. will cure congestive heart failure
   d. decrease the production of proteins by the body
   e. none of the answers are correct

5. Energy substrate solutions can be all of the following except _____ .

   a. alcohol in dextrose
   b. dextrose in water
   c. fat emulsion in water
   d. dextrose in sodium chloride
   e. fat emulsions

6. Dextrose solutions _____ .

   a. are contraindicated in patients with diabetic coma and with high blood sugar levels
   b. are used cautiously in patients receiving a corticosteroid
   c. are incompatible with blood
   d. can be in a concentrated form
   e. all of the answers are correct

7. Hetastarch may cause _____ .

   a. vomiting
   b. diarrhea
   c. blurred vision
   d. seizures
   e. ototoxicity

8. Plasma expanders are contraindicated in all of the following patients except those with _____ .

   a. severe bleeding disorders
   b. severe cardiac failure
   c. Parkinson's disease
   d. renal failure with oliguria
   e. renal failure with anuria

9. Intravenous replacement solutions _____ .

   a. are a source of electrolytes
   b. are a source of water
   c. are used to facilitate amino acid utilization
   d. maintain electrolyte balance
   e. all of the answers are correct

10. Pedialyte _____ .

    a. contains carbohydrates and electrolytes
    b. is an oral electrolyte solution
    c. is used to treat severe vomiting or diarrhea
    d. replaces lost electrolytes, carbohydrates, and fluids
    e. all of the answers are correct

11. Total parenteral nutrition is used to _____ .

    a. prevent weight loss
    b. prevent nitrogen loss
    c. treat negative nitrogen balance
    d. answers b and c are correct
    e. all of the answers are correct

12. A hyperglycemic reaction to total parenteral nutrition may be dealt with by _____ .

    a. decreasing the rate of administration
    b. reducing the dextrose concentration
    c. administering insulin
    d. all of the answers are correct
    e. none of the answers are correct

VII. RECALL FACTS

Indicate which of the following statements are Facts with an F. If the statement is not a fact, leave the line blank.

About Patient Management Issues with Electrolyte Therapy

_____ 1. Bicarbonate is used to treat respiratory acidosis.

_____ 2. Systemic overloading of calcium can cause weakness, lethargy, severe nausea and vomiting, and coma.

_____ 3. Potassium is irritating to tissues.

_____ 4. Patients receiving magnesium sulfate must be observed constantly.

_____ 5. Intravenous sodium chloride solutions can cause pulmonary edema.

_____ 6. Oral sodium bicarbonate should be taken with milk.

_____ 7. Oral potassium tablets should be chewed.

_____ 8. Direct intravenous injection of potassium can result in sudden death.

_____ 9. Magnesium sulfate can be given intramuscularly or intravenously.

_____ 10. Older adults should receive a standard dose of magnesium; only children receive a lower dose.

VIII. FILL IN THE BLANK

Fill in the blanks using words from the list below.

total parenteral nutrition   electrolytes
plasma expanders   fat emulsion
plasma protein fractions   fluid overload

1. _____ include human plasma
   protein fraction and normal serum albumin.

2. An intravenous _____ contains
   soybean or safflower oil and a mixture of natural triglycerides.

3. _____ are used to expand
   plasma volume.

4. A common adverse reaction to all solutions administered by the parenteral route is
   _____ .

5. Some _____ may cause cardiac
   irregularities.

6. _____ may be administered
   through a peripheral vein or through a central
   venous catheter.

IX. LIST

List the requested number of items.

1. List three functions of the albumin fraction of
   human blood.

   a. _____

   b. _____

   c. _____

2. List five conditions in which plasma proteins
   are contraindicated.

   a. _____

   b. _____

   c. _____

   d. _____

   e. _____

3. List the two most common adverse reactions associated with the administration of fat emulsions.

   a. _____

   b. _____

4. List three intravenous solutions of plasma expanders.

   a. _____

   b. _____

   c. _____

5. List four uses of calcium.

   a. _____

   b. _____

   c. _____

   d. _____

6. List five examples of combined intravenous electrolyte solutions.

   a. _____

   b. _____

   c. _____

   d. _____

   e. _____

7. List five products that can be used to meet the
   intravenous nutritional requirements of a patient.

   a. _____

   b. _____

   c. _____

   d. _____

   e. _____

8. List five symptoms of fluid overload.

   a. _____

   b. _____

   c. _____

   d. _____

   e. _____

9. List five conditions when TPN may be used.

a. _____

b. _____

c. _____

d. _____

e. _____

X. CLINICAL APPLICATION

1. Mr. Q's son has had a significant abdominal injury, and the trauma has disrupted his gastrointestinal system. The healthcare provider in charge of his case is planning to start him on total parenteral nutrition through a central venous line. Explain to Mr. Q why this is necessary for his son's nutritional well-being and what metabolic reactions can occur as a result of this therapy.